www.harcourt-international.com

Bringing you products from all Harcourt Health Sciences companies including Baillière Tindall, Churchill Livingstone, Mosby and W.B. Saunders

- ▶ **Browse** for latest information on new books, journals and electronic products

- ▶ **Search** for information on over 20 000 published titles with full product information including tables of contents and sample chapters

- ▶ **Keep up to date** with our extensive publishing programme in your field by registering with **eAlert** or requesting postal updates

- ▶ **Secure online ordering** with prompt delivery, as well as full contact details to order by phone, fax or post

- ▶ **News** of special features and promotions

If you are based in the following countries, please visit the country-specific site to receive full details of product availability and local ordering information

USA: www.harcourthealth.com

Canada: www.harcourtcanada.com

Australia: www.harcourt.com.au

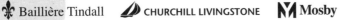 Baillière Tindall CHURCHILL LIVINGSTONE 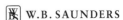 Mosby W.B. SAUNDERS

Acupuncture in the Treatment of Depression

To our families

For Churchill Livingstone

Publishing Manager: Inta Ozols
Project Development Manager: Martina Paul
Project Manager: Jane Dingwall
Design Direction: George Ajayi

Acupuncture in the Treatment of Depression

A Manual for Practice and Research

Rosa N Schnyer DiplAc
Senior Research Associate,
College of Social and Behavioral Sciences, Department of Psychology,
University of Arizona, Tucson, Arizona, USA

John J B Allen PhD
Associate Professor,
College of Social and Behavioral Sciences, Department of Psychology,
University of Arizona, Tucson, Arizona, USA

Sabrina K Hitt PhD
Research Associate,
College of Social and Behavioral Sciences, Department of Psychology,
University of Arizona, Tucson, Arizona, USA

Rachel Manber PhD
Assistant Professor,
Department of Psychiatry, University of Stanford, Stanford, California, USA

Forewords by

Ted J Kaptchuck OMD
Assistant Professor of Medicine, Harvard Medical School, Boston, Massachusetts, USA

Michael E Thase MD
Professor of Psychiatry, University of Pittsburgh School of Medicine, Pittsburgh, Pennsylvania, USA

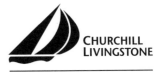

CHURCHILL
LIVINGSTONE

Edinburgh London New York Philadelphia St Louis Sydney Toronto 2001

CHURCHILL LIVINGSTONE
An imprint of Harcourt Publishers Limited

First published 2001

ISBN 0 443 07131 4

British Library Cataloguing in Publication Data
A catalogue record for this book is available from the British Library

Library of Congress Cataloging in Publication Data
A catalog record for this book is available from the Library of Congress

Note
Medical knowledge is constantly changing. As new information becomes available, changes in treatment, procedures, equipment and the use of drugs become necessary. The authors and the publishers have taken care to ensure that the information given in this text is accurate and up to date. However, readers are strongly advised to confirm that the information, especially with regard to drug usage, complies with the latest legislation and standards of practice.

The
publisher's
policy is to use
paper manufactured
from sustainable forests

Printed in China

Contents

Huang Di asked Qi Bo this question:

> In all needling, the method is above all
> Not to miss the rooting in the Spirits.
>
> *Xue* and *mai*, *ying* and *qi*, *jing*, *shen*,
> This is what the 5 *zang* store.
>
> If a situation arises
> Where, following overflowing and complete invasion,
> They leave the *zang*,
> Then the Essences are lost;
> Both *hun* and *po* are carried away in an uncontrollable agitation,
> Will and purpose become confused and disordered,
> Know-how and Reflection abandon us.
>
> Where does this state come from?
> Should one accuse Heaven? Is it the fault of Man?
>
> And what does one call Virtue, Breaths, Life, Essences, *shen*, *hun*, *po*,
> Heart, Purpose, Will, Thought, Know-how, Reflection?

Qi Bo replied:

> Heaven in me is Virtue.
> Earth in me is Breaths.
> Virtue flows. Breaths spread out, and there is Life.
> That living beings arise denotes the Essences.
> That the Essences embrace denotes the Spirits.
> That which faithfully follows the Spirits in their coming and going
>   denotes the *hun*.
> That which associates with the Essences in their exits and entries denotes
>   the *po*.
> For that which takes charge of the beings, one speaks of the Heart.
> When the Heart is applied, one speaks of Purpose.
> When Purpose is permanent, one speaks of Will.
> When Will, which is maintained, changes, one speaks of Thought.
> When Thought spreads far and powerfully, one speaks of Reflection.
> When Reflection is available to all beings, one speaks of Know-how.
> Thus Know-how is what maintains your life.
>
> Not failing to observe the Four Seasons
> And adapting to cold and heat,
> Harmonizing elation and anger
> And being calm at rest as in action,
> Regulating *yin yang*
> And balancing the hard and soft.
>
> In this way, having removed perverse influences,
> There will be long life and lasting vision...

Lingshu, Chapter 8
(Translated by Claude Larre & Elisabeth Rochat de la Vallée, 1991a)

List of Illustrations

List of Tables

Acknowledgments

Many people and organizations have been instrumental in making it possible to conduct controlled research in acupuncture and depression, and in making it possible to write this treatment manual. We first extend our gratitude to the National Institutes of Health for providing the opportunity to conduct research in alternative medicine, and for us to examine acupuncture in depression in particular (via grant numbers R21RR094921, R01MH56965 and R01AT0001, 1RO1HSO9988). We also thank the many people within the Department of Psychology at the University of Arizona for their support of our work. We would like to thank the many acupuncturists, psychologists, psychology graduate students, and psychology undergraduate students who have assisted in so many important ways. Additionally, we would like to thank Andrea Chambers for her dedicated and inexhaustible help, Leslie McGee and Cathy Travis for their invaluable contributions, and Varda Shoham for her encouragement and advice in the original study. We thank John Rush for his clarity and guidance, Mark Seem for his permission to adapt Figures 3.1 and 3.2, and his inspiration always to speak one's voice, Giovanni Maciocia for the contribution he has made to the treatment of mental–emotional disorders with acupuncture, Nigel Wiseman and Feng Ye for providing an essential resource with their dictionary of Chinese medicine, and Paul Hougham for his insightful comments. We would like to thank, especially, Bob Flaws and Blue Poppy Press for their generous permission to adapt a great deal of material from Bob's writings, including the section on menstrual disorders, disease mechanisms, patterns and treatment principles, and the sections on pregnancy and aging. Truly, Bob Flaws has been instrumental in bringing our protocol to the highest standards of the acupuncture profession. And, finally, we are grateful to all our patients and study participants; you have been the source of our encouragement and inspiration.

Forewords

The encounter of Eastern and Western medical traditions has been moving at a fast pace. Talk about "integrated" and "complementary" medicine may speak to a tendency for hasty co-habitation that may not allow for careful reflection and clear articulation of essential principles. In the industrial nations, Western medicine (a.k.a. biomedicine) is a huge edifice compared to the tiny infrastructure East Asian medicine has begun to build. This imbalance in power poses a possible danger that any partnership may mean a devaluation or dismissal of East Asian medicine's own epistemological and philosophic center of gravity. This disregard could come from either the Western or Eastern side of the encounter and becomes especially evident when scientific research requires rigid methods that may undercut the essential flexibility of Chinese medicine.

Rosa Schnyer and John Allen's new book, *Acupuncture in the Treatment of Depression*, is an ambitious attempt to create a cross-cultural medical dialogue where both sides are given sufficient time and respect to create honest partnership. This unique book actually allows both sides of a paradigmatic gulf to present their perspective and see where there are possibilities for genuine co-operation and mutual development. This collaboration even extends to the difficult terrain of allowing a traditional and realistic approach of acupuncture to be tested within the narrow confines of randomized controlled trials.

The book is an open and honest encounter. Both sides learn about the 'other' and clarify their own self-perceptions. The book's first move is biomedical: the Western nosological category of depression is explained. Then, the Chinese side presents its response to this Western description of the phenomenon. The discussion is clear, straightforward and uninterrupted. There is no rhetoric. While each side learns about the 'other,' the more important process of sharpening self-awareness is also ongoing. A psychologist will benefit from reading the Western presentation as will an acupuncturist benefit from the discussion of Chinese medicine. The Chinese medicine material presented here is a subtle, complex, valuable and undogmatic perspective that brings together many of the styles available to Western practitioners. In many ways, this discussion of acupuncture is totally refreshing and marks a milestone in our profession's ability to synthesize available approaches. Even the most veteran practitioner will benefit from this uniquely refined discussion.

The book then moves towards a collaborative understanding that would allow Chinese approaches for treating depression to be evaluated by conventional methodologies of clinical research. Each side seems ready to honor the other. Acupuncturists require flexibility, ability to treat the whole person and recognition of the legitimacy of Chinese diagnostic categories for selecting treatment. Western researchers need reproducibility, standardization, randomization and blind assessment. All these requirements are explained clearly. Both sides listen. While each side makes some compromises, the authenticity of both sides remains undiminished. A new synthesis is created and one can even speak of a new era of responsible and honest relationship between Chinese medicine and biomedicine.

Ultimately, this book is one of the very few books on Eastern and Western medicine that embodies the sensibility that Martin Buber describes in *I and Thou*: 'all real living is meeting.'

Massachusetts 2001   Ted Kaptchuk

Acupuncture is an ancient, comprehensive approach to therapeutics – it has been practiced in China for at least 5 thousand years. Acupuncture is practiced today much like it was described by Yu Hsiung in the Nei Ching (translation: Canon of Medicine), 2600 years before the birth of Jesus Christ. Acupuncture also is not new to the 'West,' as it was first exported to Europe in the 17th century. Such longevity is remarkable and may be viewed as indirect support for the belief that acupuncture has some therapeutic benefits. It is past time to learn what conditions specifically respond to acupuncture.

This book represents a serious effort to facilitate the scientific evaluation of acupuncture as a treatment for major depressive disorder. Evidence that acupuncture is an effective treatment for depression largely stems from centuries of experience treating neurasthenia, a Chinese cultural equivalent of mood disorders, as well as a handful of more recent studies.

The significance of a new, empirically verified treatment for depression should not be minimized. Major depressive disorder is a common and heterogeneous condition, which may have a lifetime incidence of up to 10% for men and 20% for women now living in the United States. Despite such a high prevalence, major depressive disorder can have devastating effects on the life of the afflicted and their significant others. In fact, the World Health Organization now considers depression to be the fourth greatest global health problem. Some evidence indicates that the age of onset of an initial depressive episode has decreased and the lifetime incidence has actually increased during the twentieth century. There is no reason to expect this pattern to change in the foreseeable future.

At the outset of the 21st century, there are already many forms of treatment known to benefit people suffering from depression. These treatments range from bright, full-spectrum in lights (at least for seasonal pattern or recurrent winter depressions) to various problem focused psychotherapies, and from a wide range of medications that affect (directly or indirectly) brain monoamine systems to electroconvulsive therapy (ECT). All treatments capitalize on nonspecific or placebo-expectancy factors, which can account for 50% to 75% of the 'action' of a proven therapy. No treatment of proven value is universally effective. A trial of antidepressant medications or focused psychotherapy will help no more than 40% to 60% of those who begin treatment. ECT nonresponse rates typically range from 20% to 40%. Perhaps as many as 10% to 20% of those who receive conventional therapy will not respond to multiple interventions and develop chronic or treatment-resistant depressive syndromes. Alternate therapies are needed for those who do not respond to, or who cannot tolerate conventional treatment.

I have spent most of my entire adult life studying the pathophysiology, diagnosis, and treatment of mood disorders, including the various forms of depression and bipolar disorder. The Western approach to psychiatric medicine, in which I am thoroughly entrenched, is anchored in the scientific method. We view this approach as an inherently superior system of obtaining knowledge. Nevertheless, the 'truths' of one moment not uncommonly require revision within the next 10 to 20 years.

The notion that acupuncture may be an effective 'antidepressant' will be provocative to most American and European mental health professionals. The theoretical basis for treatment efficacy described by Schnyer and colleagues is not unlike the humoral models of Hippocrates or Galen, yet 'theory derived' remedies such as dunking, bleeding, and warm woolen 'rubs' have long ceased to be part of the Western approach to treatment of depression. It is always humbling to recall the story of Dr Ignaz Semmelweis, who was essentially run out of nineteenth-century Vienna for his provocative suggestion that obstetricians should scrub their hands between deliveries and examination. Most of Semmelweis's contemporaries thought he was a fool because his work predated 'germ theory' by about 20 years.

Does acupuncture really have antidepressant effects over and above its substantial capacity to mobilize expectancy and other nonspecific factors? Only time (and the results of properly controlled clinical trials) will tell. The randomized clinical trial was not part of the paradigm of traditional Chinese medicine and, until recently, the cadre of Western investigators able to conduct such studies have not been interested in evaluating complementary or alternative treatments. The studies that have been done, including a pilot study by the authors, are either small or in other cases poorly standardized. But, although the evidence base for acupuncture lags far behind pharmacotherapy, is not too far behind that of psychodynamic psychotherapy!

If acupuncture does have therapeutic effects, are they really the result of reversal of qi stagnation or altered blood vacuity? Of course not. The theoretic models of Yu Hsiung were not informed by knowledge of functional neuroanatomy or neurophysiology and are bound to the ways of knowing that defined the time and place that shaped the work. But, Qi stagnation is not much more than aggression turned inward. Moreover, the early hypotheses about the mechanisms of action of electroconvulsive therapy or antidepressants are no longer credible.

The demonstration of efficacy will oblige us to examine the contributions of ascending peripheral and visceral inputs in the maintenance of emotional 'tone', neurovegetative processes such as sleep and appetite, and central nervous system stress response syndromes. The neurobiological paradigms that will enable investigators to trace the impact of therapeutic needling to key neural circuits involving the brain stem, limbic system, and prefrontal cortex are now available. Ultimately, the methods to ascertain the effects of acupuncture on gene activity similarly will be on line.

Publication of a treatment manual for acupuncture permits the key 'abilities' of the scientific method to be mobilized – operationalizabilty, testability, refutability, and replicability. The authors are to be congratulated for their hard work and willingness to swim against the current of contemporary pharmacologic and psychotherapeutic hegemonies. After centuries of mystery, things could happen quickly!

Pennsylvania 2001   Michael E. Thase

Preface

In response to US Congressional legislation in 1991 sponsored by Senator Tom Harkin (D-Iowa), the Office of Alternative Medicine (OAM) was established within the National Institutes of Health (NIH) during the Federal Government's 1992 Fiscal Year. The OAM was charged with evaluating what was then termed 'unconventional medical practices' and has been more recently and less pejoratively relabeled 'Alternative Medicine'. The purpose of the OAM 'is to encourage the investigation of alternative medical practices, with the ultimate goal of integrating validated alternative medical practices with conventional medical procedures' (RFA OD-93-002).

In March 1993, the OAM issued a Request for Applications (RFA) that was designed to encourage collaborations between conventional researchers and practitioners of alternative medicine to conduct small-scale studies to collect preliminary data concerning the evaluation of alternative medicine. The response to the RFA exceeded all expectations, with over 400 grant applications submitted. After a peer-review process by committees comprised of conventional researchers as well as those versed in alternative medicine, 30 NIH Exploratory/Development Grants (R21) were awarded, each of which did not exceed a total cost of $30,000. By conventional standards, these were very small grants. On the other hand, never before in NIH history had alternative medicine been supported to such a degree.

In response to this RFA, we (the authors of this book) collaborated to propose an acupuncture treatment study of major depression in women. Our interest in this grant stemmed from the first author's clinical experience with depressive symptoms in her clients, and from the second author's research interests in risk for depression. Through an interactive writing process, we learned to speak one another's language – learning that sound scientific research need not be incompatible with a flexible individually tailored acupuncture treatment approach. To our delight, our proposal was among the 30 funded proposals and, along with one other proposal, the only proposal to study acupuncture. The results of our study, for which a prototype of this treatment manual was used, are summarized briefly in Chapter 7 of this manual.

Since the first round of small R21 grants, the OAM has awarded another dozen small grants, and also several larger grants given to centers for research in alternative medicine. It was intended that the recipients of the original small grants would submit follow-up research proposals to conventional NIH programs. From our perspective, the original OAM grant initiative achieved its mission: it provided us with the opportunity to gather preliminary data that can form the basis of a larger research effort. We believe that research on alternative medicine can and should compete at the same level as research on conventional methods. At the same time, we must acknowledge that there may exist a reluctance by conventional researchers to view alternative medicine as worthy of scientific investigation or research funding (see *New York Times*, June 18, 1996).

Since its inception, the OAM has gone through two transformations. The first involved renaming the OAM as the Office of Complementary and Alternative Medicine, in recognition of the growing role for alternative treatments to be used in conjunction with 'established' treatments. The second transformation involved promoting this office to become the National Center for Complementary and Alternative Medicine (NCCAM), allowing this center to control funding directly just as the other National Institutes of Health divisions. The Congressional mandate establishing the NCCAM stated that the Center's purpose is to 'facilitate the evaluation of alternative medical treatment modalities' to determine their effectiveness, and also to provide for a public information clearinghouse and a research training program. The mandate also increased the budget of this office from $20 million to $50 million.

It is an exciting time to be involved in research on alternative medicine. As research in alternative and complementary treatments increases in response to the NCCAM growth, there will be the need for well-detailed treatment approaches that can be implemented in different research settings as well as in everyday practice. This treatment manual was created in the hope of providing such a research protocol in which therapies are reproducible, yet individually tailored. Moreover, it was created to make available to the acupuncturist practitioner a well-delineated assessment and treatment framework.

If we wish to find an answer, we must first ask the proper question. If we wish to ask the proper question, we must first formulate it explicitly. It is our hope that this book moves us one step closer in this journey of inquiry.

Rosa N Schnyer
John J B Allen

Arizona 2001

1 **Background and Context**

INTRODUCTION

Although acupuncture has been practiced for over 3000 years (Ulett 1992), the Western psychological and psychiatric scientific community has produced little empirical research on the efficacy of acupuncture. With the notable exception of acupuncture as a treatment for substance abuse and dependence (for reviews see Brewington et al 1994, McLellan et al 1993), there are very few well-controlled empirical studies of the efficacy of acupuncture for psychiatric disorders. The need for empirical trials is underscored by recent surveys documenting the popularity of alternative treatments for psychiatric and emotional disorders (Cassidy 1998, Eisenberg et al 1993, 1998).

This book is written in the hope of articulating how the traditional principles on which acupuncture is based can be applied to the treatment of psychiatric problems. It is written for clinical practitioners of acupuncture, for researchers, and for other healthcare providers interested in learning about the potential use of acupuncture in the area of mental health. This book is designed to provide a standardized framework for the assessment of depressive symptoms from the perspective of Chinese Medicine (CM) and a manualized approach to devising treatment plans that are individually tailored to address each individual's constellation of signs and symptoms. It may be helpful to clarify that throughout this text the term standardization is used when refer-

Parts of this chapter appear in Schnyer & Allen (2001) and are included here with the permission of the publisher, WB Saunders.

ring to the standardization of the methodology employed in assessment and treatment design – in this case primarily the eight guiding criteria – to emphasize the selection of a specific framework. It should be differentiated from the current trend towards standardizing the practice of Chinese Medicine to reflect exclusively the traditional (TCM) model (Fruehauf 1999). The approach presented in this book is not intended to serve as the sole and definitive approach to the clinical treatment of depression with acupuncture. The field of Chinese Medicine continues to grow precisely because of the rich diversity of clinical approaches that characterize the profession. It is hoped that this book can serve as a model and offer inspiration for other acupuncture traditions; the advancement of our profession will depend on making it amenable to scientific inquiry, which has become the 'gold standard' for evaluating treatments and making policy decisions.

It is intended that this manual will not only facilitate research, but also open the opportunity for acupuncture practitioners to implement a manualized treatment approach in their own practice. The benefits of using such a manualized approach are many, but include: (1) greater systematic attention to detail, (2) the opportunity to implement an experimentally tested protocol in routine clinical practice, and (3) the opportunity to gather data on the effectiveness of a researched approach in the real world setting of clinical practice.

The approach taken in this manual follows from standard principles of Chinese Medicine, which are described in detail in standard texts such as *The Web That Has No Weaver: Understanding Chinese Medicine* (Kaptchuk 1983), *The Practice of Chinese Medicine* (Maciocia 1994), *The Foundations of Chinese Medicine* (Maciocia 1989), and *A Compendium of Traditional Chinese Medicine Patterns and Treatment* (Flaws & Finney 1996). The manual is designed for use with persons that meet Western criteria for major depression (see Ch. 2) of less than 2 years' duration, according to the diagnostic criteria of the *Diagnostic and Statistical Manual*, fourth edition (DSM-IV; American Psychiatric Association 1994).

ESSENTIAL FEATURES OF THE APPROACH

The features of the approach in this manual should be familiar to any practitioner trained in Chinese Medicine:

- An assumption that Western-defined depression is heterogeneous and may be characterized by one or more distinct patterns of disharmony, which may differ for different clients with depression.

- Differential diagnosis using signs and symptoms, client interview, taking of pulses, and an examination of the tongue, integrating five areas:
  - eight principles
  - qi, blood and body fluids
  - viscera and bowels
  - channels and network vessels
  - five phases.

- Given a pattern of disharmony or combination of patterns identified through differential diagnosis, the development of specific treatment principles.

- The selection of points to address the treatment principles.

- Acute treatments delivered twice per week for 8 weeks, and once per week for 4 weeks.

- Maintenance and continuation treatments semimonthly and then monthly for the next year.

- A goal of producing clinically meaningful change: improved balance rather than disharmony, remission as defined by DSM-IV criteria, and Hamilton Rating Scale for Depression (HRSD) score ≤ 6.

Moreover, this manual details assessment and treatment suitable for persons with DSM-IV-defined major depression of less than 2 years' duration. The details of diagnosing major depression are covered in Chapter 2. It is not necessarily the case that the framework and techniques in this manual are not useful, at least in part, for people who do not meet the restricted criteria for major depression, but the effectiveness of this treatment for conditions other than narrowly defined major depression (Ch. 2) has not been investigated systematically. Moreover, although the approach has been tested with women, it is currently being tested with men. In addition, the approach remains untested with clients with comorbid disorders, dysthymia, and chronic depression (see Ch. 2). Finally, although it is the authors' view that acupuncture can be fruitfully combined with psychotherapy, this manual covers the use of acupuncture as the exclusive treatment, without adjunct treatments such as psychotherapy, pharmacotherapy, or herbal interventions.

A COMMENT ON THE INTEGRATION OF SCIENTIFIC RESEARCH AND CHINESE MEDICINE

This book was written with the aim of promoting sound scientific research on acupuncture and depression, while still providing flexibility and individualization in assessment and treatment planning – a necessary feature of Chinese Medicine. The theoretical paradigms that underlie acupuncture are very different from the Western medical models. Therefore, proper research studies in this field must incorporate an energetic diagnosis based on the principles of Chinese Medicine (CM) in order to identify treatment protocols correctly, rather than rely solely on Western diagnostic systems (Bensoussan 1990).

The utilization of a manualized treatment approach in clinical trials involving acupuncture provides the essential flexibility necessary to deliver individualized treatment, while conforming to the standardization fundamental to conducting sound research. The use of a treatment manual promotes the systematic articulation of the chosen framework (in this case primarily the eight principles), thus providing replicability and systematization while allowing for individualized treatment. Additionally, a manualized treatment approach increases the quality and consistency of the treatment by standardizing the technical aspects, providing a precise framework for training and supervision, enabling the evaluation of practitioner competence and conformity, and increasing the ability to identify the most essential therapeutic aspects of the approach. A treatment manual should not aim at limiting treatment options within a narrowly defined protocol, but rather it should provide the freedom to identify a variety of treatment possibilities within a sound conceptual framework.

According to Chinese Medicine, any piece of information (symptom or sign) gathered from the client can be interpreted only in relation to other symptoms and signs. The integration and consideration of all significant variables that relate to the process of diagnosis and treatment is paramount in Chinese Medicine. Rather than eliminate variables in order to control the treatment outcome, Chinese Medicine seeks to integrate all significant variables, in order to create the most effective treatment. A certain flexibility is needed to assess accurately the efficacy of acupuncture, precisely because the theory of acupuncture is structured around the integration of data. Nevertheless, some standardization of treatment is necessary for the purposes of replication in research and clinical practice (Bensoussan 1990).

In other words, individuals who share a Western diagnosis (e.g. depression) will be characterized by a variety of CM-based *patterns of disharmony* which, in turn, dictate particular treatments to address these patterns of disharmony. Treatments, therefore, must be tailored to each individual's symptom picture; a 'standard' treatment must not be uniformly administered to all individuals who share a Western diagnosis. This manual describes the framework and procedures by which acupuncturists may reliably arrive at individualized diagnoses and treatment plans. In pilot work designed specifically to assess how

well individuals could agree using this framework and these procedures, five women with major depression were seen independently by
two acupuncturists within a 3-day period. Overall agreement was
quite high, as indicated by an intraclass correlation coefficient[1] of
0.78, summarizing their composite agreement. This result suggests
that practitioners can agree on which pattern(s) of disharmony characterize any given individual's depression, and agree on the treatment
that should ensue.

PREVIOUS RESEARCH

Aside from our pilot study (Allen et al 1998), which is detailed in
Chapter 7, the only studies of acupuncture as a treatment for depression or depression-like syndromes have been published in China
(Chengying 1992, Han 1986) and in Eastern Europe and the former
Soviet Union (Cherkezova & Toteva 1991, Frydrychowski et al 1984,
Polyakov & Dudaeva 1990, Polyakov 1987, 1988). It is difficult to
evaluate these studies fully, because the diagnostic criteria used differ
from those of the DSM-IV, and because most of these studies have not
been translated into English (other than the abstracts). Collectively,
however, these studies suggest that acupuncture may be effective in
the treatment of depression and depressive symptoms, in some cases
as effective as tricyclic antidepressant medication. The following
review summarizes these studies, with a focus on the range of depressive symptoms for which acupuncture may and may not be effective.

Polyakov (1988) treated 167 depressed patients with acupuncture.
Acupuncture reduced the principal symptoms of depression and also
lessened the severity and prominence of supplementary symptoms.
The best results from acupuncture were obtained in patients with
melancholic depression; poor results were obtained in patients with
anxious and apathetic depressions. Acupuncture was almost as effective as antidepressants in cyclothymic depressions and was notably
inferior to tricyclic antidepressants in patients with psychotic features.
Moreover, Polyakov (1988) reported that follow-up studies over 1–2
years indicated that adequate maintenance therapy produces results
comparable to drug therapy, although inadequate information was
provided to evaluate this claim. In this study, acupuncture was carried
out using a standardized method of treatment that consisted of five
acupuncture points located in the traditional meridians (St 36, P 5,
P 6, Lu 7, and LI 4) plus three ear acupuncture points (AT affect,

---

[1]The intraclass correlation ranges from 0 (no agreement) to 1 (perfect agreement). Diagnostic
instruments typically will have values greater than 0.7 on this statistic.

AT Shen-men, and AT Zero). From the perspective of pattern differential diagnosis (the assessment method of Chinese Medicine), the finding of poor treatment response in anxious and apathetic depressions is not surprising, because this set of points does not specifically address the features present during anxious or apathetic depressions. This highlights the importance of considering individual differences in symptom presentation and tailoring points accordingly, as detailed in this manual.

Other studies provide only abstracts in English. Chengying (1992) used points on the Du channel (which runs along the spine) to treat a mélange of psychiatric disorders including anxiety, depression, hypochondria, neurasthenia, obsessive–compulsive disorder, aphasia, alexia, and hysterical paralysis. A total of 115 patients with a course of disease from 2 months to 8 years were treated with points selected from the Du channel. Points were selected by pressing the points one by one, observing and comparing sensitivity to the points, and choosing to needle the 1–2 points with the maximum response. Of the 115 patients, 61 experienced complete disappearance of psychoneurotic and somatic symptoms and no recurrence at 6-month follow-up, 31 experienced a significant improvement, and 23 had no significant improvement after treatment. Although Chenying (1992) studied a heterogeneous group, the comparability of the diagnoses neurasthenia and major depression was noted by Chang (1984). Commenting on the observations of Dunner & Dunner (1983), Chang indicated that almost 50% of psychiatric outpatients in China are diagnosed with neurasthenia, and that many of these neurasthenics would be diagnosed by the DSM with major depression. Moreover, Chang (1984) noted that antidepressants were as effective with cases of neurasthenia diagnosed by Chinese psychiatrists as with cases of DSM-defined depression.

A further 103 patients with neurasthenia (course of disease from 3 months to 20 years, average of 4.5 years) were observed clinically at the Academy of Traditional Chinese Medicine (Suobin 1991). Principal points Du 14, Du 13, GB 20, the first line on the Bladder channel, bilateral to the spine and the Huatuo paravertebral points (M BW 35 (Jiaji); O'Connor & Bensky 1981) were used, along with other points chosen according to symptoms. Following treatment 45 patients were relieved of all their symptoms and were considered clinically cured, 29 experienced an improvement of the main symptoms but some secondary symptoms remained, 21 experienced a noticeable improvement, and eight had no improvement at all.

Another Chinese study, by Luo, Jia, and Zhan of the Institute of Mental Health, Beijing Medical College, examined electroacupuncture and amitriptyline treatment of DSM-III-defined major depression. This study, summarized by Han (1986), found comparable decreases in HRSD scores as a function of electroacupuncture and amitriptyline treatments over a 5-week interval: mean ± SD HRSD scores dropped from 28.5 ± 1.2 to 12.8 ± 2.0 for patients receiving acupuncture, and from 29.4 ± 1.4 to 14.2 ± 1.9 for those receiving amitriptyline. Moreover, fewer side effects were reported for patients receiving electroacupuncture. Unfortunately, this study used only two points (Du 20 and Yintang), and it is unclear whether standard needling, as opposed to *electro*acupuncture, would provide comparable results, although some (Ulett 1992) claim that the effect of acupuncture is due entirely to the frequency of stimulation rather than to the specific points selected. Another Chinese study (Hechun 1988; summarized by Brewington et al 1994) also found comparable decreases in depressive symptoms in patients having electroacupuncture and those receiving amitriptyline. Finally, acupuncture also appears to diminish depressive symptoms in the context of opiate detoxification (Cherkezova & Toteva 1991, Newmeyer et al 1984).

Although far from definitive, taken together these studies suggest that it is possible to obtain favorable results using acupuncture to treat mood-related symptoms, including depression. These findings encouraged us to undertake a pilot study to examine the efficacy of acupuncture as a treatment for depression. To undertake such a study, we devised this manual to ensure that a standardized treatment approach would be used. Chapters 3 and 4 detail the framework of Chinese Medicine that underlies our approach, and Chapter 5 presents the details of the application of this approach. Chapter 6 then presents the results of several case studies viewed in light of the treatment approach. Chapter 7 discusses research methods, and concludes with the presentation of results from our pilot study using this treatment approach. Chapters 8 and 9 of the manual describe clinical applications, and these chapters attempt to suggest ways in which the approach may be extended for use in settings other than those in which it has been explicitly investigated. In Chapter 10 we offer our conclusions.

2 Depression Defined: Symptoms, Epidemiology, Etiology, and Treatment

INTRODUCTION

Depression is a term that has been used to describe a variety of ailments, ranging from minor to incapacitating. Clinically significant depression, termed major depression, is a serious condition characterized not only by depressed mood, but a cluster of somatic, cognitive, and motivational symptoms. Major depression can be differentiated from a normal and transient sad mood by several factors:

- intensity, as major depression causes impairment in social or occupational functioning and persists across time and situations

- relationship to antecedent events, as major depression either occurs without any identifiable antecedent event or is clearly in excess of what would be considered an expected reaction

- quality, with the quality of the emotion being different from that experienced in a normal sad mood

- associated features, as the mood co-occurs with a group of other cognitive and somatic symptoms

- history, with major depression typically appearing after a history of other such episodes (Whybrow et al 1984).

Individuals who are suffering from major depression often report feeling overwhelmed, helpless, despairing, suffocated, or numb. Major depression can range from mild sadness to complete hopelessness and is often accompanied by frequent crying spells. Those with more severe depression may feel like crying but be unable to do so. Severely depressed individuals often believe that no one can help them.

Depression is defined according to specific criteria outlined in the Diagnostic and Statistical Manual of Mental Disorders, fourth edition (DSM-IV) (American Psychiatric Association (APA) 1994).[1]

The DSM-IV details the diagnostic criteria for nearly 300 mental disorders, and nearly 100 other psychological conditions that might be the focus of professional attention. While many individuals experiencing a debilitating depression will meet criteria for one of the disorders within the DSM-IV, some will nonetheless elude classification using this system. The following sections detail the different disorders within the DSM-IV that may involve depressive symptoms, following which an overview of etiology and treatment – for the non-specialist – is provided.

MAJOR DEPRESSIVE DISORDER (MAJOR DEPRESSION)

In order to be diagnosed with a major depressive episode according to the DSM-IV, an individual must have at least five out of nine possible symptoms, which must be present during the same 2-week period and represent a change from a previous level of functioning. One of the symptoms must be either depressed mood for most of the day on nearly every day, or loss of interest or pleasure (anhedonia) in all or almost all activities for most of the day on nearly every day. Additional symptoms that may accompany the depressed mood or anhedonia are:

- significant weight loss (when not dieting) or significant weight gain (i.e. more than 5% of body weight in 1 month), or a decreased or increased appetite nearly every day

- insomnia or hypersomnia nearly every day

- observable psychomotor agitation or retardation nearly every day

- fatigue or loss of energy nearly every day, feelings of worthlessness

- or excessive or inappropriate guilt nearly every day

- diminished ability to think or concentrate, or indecisiveness nearly every day

- and recurrent thoughts of death (not just fear of dying) or suicide.

[1]Depression is also often diagnosed according to criteria outlined in the *ICD-10 Classification of Mental and Behavioral Disorders* (World Health Organization 1992). ICD-10 criteria overlap substantially, but are not identical to, those of the DSM-IV. This chapter focuses on the criteria of the DSM-IV because the studies reviewed here have predominantly relied on these criteria for diagnosing depression.

The symptoms must be present for at least 2 weeks and cause clinically significant distress or impairment in social, occupational, or other areas of functioning. Additionally the mood disturbance should not be the direct physiological effect of a substance (e.g. street drug or medication) or general medical condition (e.g. hypothyroidism) (APA 1994). Individuals who meet criteria for a major depressive episode and have never experienced any manic or hypomanic episodes (see below) then meet criteria for major depressive disorder.

Unipolar Versus Bipolar Depression

The DSM-IV distinguishes two broad classes of mood disorder: unipolar and bipolar disorder. Unipolar disorders involve only the depressed dimension of mood and do not include periods of above-average mood such as manic or hypomanic episodes. There are two unipolar mood disorders: major depressive disorder and dysthymic disorder. Bipolar disorders include those in which the individual experiences both depressed moods and manic or hypomanic episodes. The three bipolar disorders described in DSM-IV are bipolar I disorder, bipolar II disorder, and cyclothymic disorder.

Dysthymia

Another form of depression that is less intense but more chronic than major depressive disorder is dysthymia. Distinguishing between a diagnosis of major depressive disorder and dysthymia is difficult because the two share many symptoms and the differences in onset, duration, persistence, and severity are difficult to evaluate retrospectively. In order to meet DSM-IV criteria for dysthymic disorder, an individual must experience depressed mood for most of the day, more days than not for at least 2 years. In children and adolescents, irritable mood would also suffice to meet the criteria, and must last for at least 1 year. Two or more additional symptoms must also be present: poor appetite or overeating, insomnia or hypersomnia, low energy or fatigue, low self-esteem, poor concentration or difficulty making decisions, and feelings of hopelessness. At no time during the 2-year period has such a person been without the depressive symptoms for more than 2 months at a time. If the person has met criteria for major depression at any point during the 2-year period, the diagnosis would be considered as major depression instead of dysthymia. However, an individual who has met criteria for dysthymia for at least 2 years and then subsequently meets the criteria for an episode of major depression superimposed on the dysthymia (without an intervening remission) would be given both diagnoses. This condition is referred to as double depression. It is particularly difficult to differentiate double depression from simple major depressive disorder or chronic major depressive disorder for the reasons mentioned above, combined with the fact that all three meet criteria for a major depressive episode and they differ only in onset, duration, and persistence. A history of mania (at least one manic episode) would rule out a diagnosis of both major depression and dysthymia (APA 1994).

Mania and Bipolar Disorder

Mania is the mood state that is the apparent opposite of depression. Mania involves a euphoric or elated mood that lasts for at least 1 week. A manic episode is more than just a normal good mood; rather, the person feels like he or she is on top of the world and there is nothing he/she can't do. The euphoric mood is accompanied by at least three other symptoms, including: inflated self-esteem or grandiose beliefs (e.g. that the patient is President or some other famous person of importance), a decreased need for sleep (i.e. feels rested after only 3 h of sleep), a pressure to keep talking, the subjective experience that one's thoughts are racing, distractibility, increase in activity (either socially, at work or school, or sexually), and excessive involvement in pleasurable activities that have a high potential for painful consequences (e.g. unrestrained buying sprees, sexual promiscuity, etc.). In addition, the mood disturbance must cause impairment in functioning (either social or occupational), or require hospitalization to prevent harm to self or others, or involve psychotic features (e.g. hallucinations). Furthermore, a manic episode is not diagnosed if the symptoms are caused by street drugs, medication or other treatment, or a general medical condition (APA 1994).

A person who has experienced at least one manic episode would meet the criteria for bipolar I disorder. Most individuals who meet criteria for bipolar I have also experienced episodes of major depression in addition to manic episodes; however, this is not necessary for the diagnosis.

Some individuals experience a mood disturbance called hypomania that is similar to a manic episode, but not as severe. The criteria for hypomania are the same as the criteria for a manic episode (described above); however, hypomania must only be present for at least 4 days (versus 1 week for a manic episode), and the episode must not cause impairment in functioning or require hospitalization. Individuals who have experienced at least one major depressive episode, at least one hypomanic episode, and no fully developed manic episodes would be give a diagnosis of bipolar II disorder (APA 1994).

Cyclothymia

Cyclothymia is a more chronic but less intense form of bipolar disorder. To meet criteria for cyclothymia, an individual must experience numerous periods of hypomania and depressed mood over a period of at least 2 years. In fact, the person cannot show the absence of both hypomanic and depressive symptoms for a period of more than 2 months. Moreover, in cyclothymia there are no major depressive episodes or manic episodes during the first 2 years of the disorder (APA 1994).

Table 2.1 summarizes the mood disorders described in this section. Although it is possible that acupuncture may prove effective in treating many varieties of depression, our previous clinical trial (Allen et al 1998) examined only major depressive disorder, and this manual is designed for use with major depressive disorder. With modifications, it is possible that the framework detailed in the subsequent chapters could be adapted for use with other depressive disorders.

TABLE 2.1	A summary of mood disorders in the diagnostic and statistical manual, fourth edition
Mood disorder	**Description**
Unipolar disorders	
Major depressive disorder	One or more major depressive episodes No manic or unequivocal hypomanic episodes
Dysthymic disorder	Depressed mood for at least 2 years Never without these symptoms for more than 2 months during this period No major depressive episodes during first 2 years
Bipolar disorders	
Bipolar I disorder	One or more manic episodes
Bipolar II disorder	One or more major depressive episodes At least one hypomanic episode No manic episodes
Cyclothymic disorder	Numerous periods with hypomanic symptoms and numerous periods with depressed mood for at least 2 years Never without these symptoms for more than 2 months during 2-year period No major depressive episodes No manic episode during first 2 years

Source: Oltmans & Emery (1995).

Specifiers of Major Depression

To capture more adequately the range of mood disorders, the DSM-IV additionally provides for the inclusion of specifiers, which can be

TABLE 2.2	Specifiers for DSM mood disorders
Specifier	**Description**
Chronic	Major depressive disorder can be categorized as chronic if the individual meets criteria continuously for 2 years or more. Individuals with chronic major depression tend to be less responsive to treatment.
Melancholic	Major depressive disorder with melancholic features is a subtype in which patients demonstrate either anhedonia or lack of reactivity to pleasurable stimuli, and more somatic symptoms (e.g. early morning awakening, weight loss, and psychomotor agitation or retardation) than in other types of depression.
Psychotic features	Major depressive disorder can be accompanied by delusions or hallucinations which are usually focused on mood-congruent depressive themes (e.g. the depression is a punishment for past errors or sinful deeds) but may be incongruent with mood (e.g. delusions about being persecuted).
Postpartum	The postpartum specifier is applied when the onset of the episode is within 4 weeks of childbirth.
Atypical	The atypical features specifier is applied when the individual experiences mood reactivity (i.e. mood improves in response to positive events).
Course Specifier	
Seasonal pattern	This is a pattern in which the depressive episodes regularly commence during a particular season, usually winter, and remit during a specific time of year (e.g. the depression ends in spring or summer). This patter of depression is frequently accompanied by symptoms such as lethargy, hypersomnia, overeating, weight gain, and carbohydrate craving. This specifier is most commonly applied to major depression but can also be used for bipolar II and less commonly bipolar I.
Rapid cycling	The course of a bipolar disorder (bipolar I or II) can be described as rapid cycling if the individual experiences at least four episodes of a major depressive, manic, or hypomanic episode within a 1-year period.

Source: American Psychiatric Association (1994).

used to describe the current or most recent major depressive episode included. These specifiers (see Table 2.2) include chronic, with melancholic features, severe with psychotic features, postpartum onset, and atypical. In addition, the course of the disorder can be specified as 'with seasonal pattern', which is considered a subtype of major depression also known as seasonal affective disorder. The bipolar disorders can be specified as rapid cycling. The DSM-IV provides additional information on the specifiers listed in Table 2.2.

Epidemiology of Major Depression

Major depression is an unfortunately common condition. Lifetime prevalence estimates vary from 5% (Robins et al 1984) to 17% in a more recent large-scale survey (Kessler et al 1994). Lifetime prevalence indexes the proportion of individuals that will contract major depression at some point during life. Unipolar depression is approximately twice as common among women as among men (Nolen-Hoeksema 1987). The 12-month prevalence of major depression is 7.7% in men and 12.9% in women, and the lifetime prevalence rate is 12% for men and 21% for women (Kessler et al 1994).

The costs of major depression are substantial, and exceed those of other chronic diseases such as diabetes and hypertension in terms of personal distress, lost productivity, interpersonal problems, and suicide. A recent study estimated that these annual costs of depression in the United States exceeded $40 billion (Hirschfeld & Schatzberg 1994), and similar findings have emerged from a worldwide study (Murry & Lopez 1996) that ranked unipolar major depression as the number one cause of disability in the world. Over 80% of individuals who committed suicide were clinically depressed in the months before their death, and the lifetime risk for suicide among those with clinical depression is 15% (Hirschfeld & Schatzberg 1994). Furthermore, depressed individuals appear to be at increased risk of death from all causes. A 16-year prospective study found that mortality rates for depressed individuals are 1.5–2 times those of nondepressed individuals (Murphy et al 1987). Clearly, depression is a prevalent disorder with costly and potentially lethal consequences (Gotlib & Beach 1995).

Comorbidity of Major Depression with other Mental Disorders

Comorbidity is the presence of two or more disorders simultaneously. Comorbid conditions are generally more chronic, do not respond as well to treatment, and have a poorer prognosis than single disorders. It is important to be aware of the issue of comorbidity because a large proportion of individuals in the general population have more than one mental disorder concurrently (Kessler et al 1994). Outcome studies usually examine efficacy for individuals with only one disorder. Therefore, the average clinician deals with much more complicated cases than outcome research addresses (Greenberg & Fisher 1997). In fact, the National Comorbidity Survey found that it was more common to have two or more mental disorders than to have only one (Kessler et al 1994).

Dysthymia is present before the onset of a major depressive disorder in approximately 10% of epidemiological samples. Other forms of mental illness may be present concurrent with major depressive disorder, such as: alcohol abuse or dependence disorder, personality disorders (e.g. borderline personality disorder), panic disorder, and other anxiety disorders (APA 1994). The literature demonstrates that 33–59% of people who are dependent on alcohol eventually meet criteria for depression at some point during the disorder (Merikangas & Gelernter 1990). The comorbidity of personality disorders in clinically depressed individuals is 50% or greater (Zimmerman et al 1991). The comorbidity of anxiety disorders with depression is particularly high, in the range of 30% (Hiller et al 1989) to 57% (Mannuzza et al 1989). Research demonstrates that between 15 and 30% of individuals with acute major depression also suffer from panic disorder concurrently (Brown & Barlow 1992). The diagnostic criteria of anxiety and depression overlap, which increases the probability of meeting criteria for both disorders simultaneously. This overlap makes it difficult to know whether there exist two separate classes of conditions – anxiety and depression – or whether there may exist a single underlying predisposition that manifests with both depression and anxiety symptoms (see Frances et al 1992). In addition, the overlap increases lifetime comorbidity (i.e. meeting criteria for both depression and an anxiety disorder) between the disorders (Klerman 1990). The comorbidity of anxiety disorders with depression poses a taxonomic enigma (see Frances et al 1992) for diagnosticians and those interested in etiology.

In addition, 20–25% of individuals with general medical conditions such as diabetes, myocardial infarction, carcinoma, and stroke meet criteria for major depressive disorder at some point during the course of their illness (APA 1994). Depression may occur in the context of medical illness for three reasons: (1) the depression appears to represent a reaction to the burden and limitations associated with having a disease, (2) the depression is unrelated to the disease, but is a recurrence of a long-standing history of depression, or is in response to some other event in the person's life, or (3) the depression occurs as a direct physiological consequence of the medical condition (e.g. multiple sclerosis, stroke, hypothyroidism). In this latter case the diagnosis is technically not major depressive disorder, but rather mood disorder due to a general medical condition. A mood disorder can also be directly etiologically related to the use of a medication or a drug of abuse. In that case a diagnosis of substance-induced mood disorder (e.g. cocaine-induced mood disorder) is made instead of major depressive disorder. However, this diagnosis is reserved for depression that is a direct physiological consequence of the drug abuse or medication use; for example, the depressed mood is only present following withdrawal from cocaine (APA 1994).

This latter determination is often difficult to make because of the high rates of comorbid substance abuse or dependence disorders and mood disorders. In some cases individuals may begin using substances in response to depression, in an unfortunate attempt to cope with their pain. In such a case, major depression would be comorbid with substance abuse, and both diagnoses would be given. In other cases, it could be that a pre-existing substance abuse disorder appeared to cause the depression through direct physiological means (e.g. cocaine withdrawal), in which case the diagnosis would be substance-induced mood disorder (see DSM-IV for further clarification of these diagnostic issues).

THE EFFICACY OF 'CONVENTIONAL' TREATMENTS FOR DEPRESSION

A variety of well-researched treatments exist for depression, and most have rather favorable results. These treatments include both psychotherapies and drug therapies. Unfortunately, however, the effectiveness of these traditional treatments is hampered by high rates of dropout, recovery failure, and relapse, suggesting that these traditional treatments may provide insufficient or transient symptom relief for many.

The National Institutes of Mental Health Treatment of Depression Collaborative Research Program was a clinical trial designed to investigate the efficacy of two brief psychotherapies (interpersonal psychotherapy and cognitive behavior therapy) and a drug treatment (pharmacotherapy with imipramine hydrochloride, a tricyclic antidepressant), all compared with a control group consisting of clinical management combined with pill-placebo as treatments for major depression. In this NIMH treatment study, 32% of patients who were randomized to treatment discontinued treatment prematurely. Excluding patients who dropped out for external reasons or because they had improved, 25% of all patients entering treatment terminated due to negative effects of the treatment such as dissatisfaction with treatment, desire for another treatment, intolerable side effects, and noncompliance (Elkin et al 1989). Among patients who had completed 15 weeks of pharmacotherapy or psychotherapy (not including the placebo group), 43–49% failed to recover to the point of having few symptoms, and among all patients including completers and non-completers 30–64% did not have significant symptom relief at the end of treatment (Elkin et al 1989).

Advocates of standard antidepressant medications (e.g. tricyclics such as imipramine) generally acknowledge that about one-third of patients do not improve with medication, one-third display improvement with placebos, and the remaining third demonstrate improvement that would not occur with placebo (Greenberg & Fisher 1997). In a meta-analysis (a statistical literature review that has compressed the results of large numbers of studies) of antidepressant outcome in which clinician bias was minimized, Greenberg et al (1992) found that effect sizes were approximately one-half to one-quarter as large as those found in previous studies in which clinician bias was not minimized. Clinician bias was reduced by examining the effectiveness of standard antidepressant tricyclic medications compared with newer antidepressants (serotonin reuptake inhibitors; SSRIs) as well as a placebo control. Presumably, in studies with such a design there is less motivation to establish the efficacy of the standard antidepressants, yet their effects can still be compared with those of a placebo control. With the advent of a new generation of antidepressants (SSRIs), it was hoped that they would be superior in treating depression to the older medications. A meta-analysis of all of the double-blind placebo-controlled efficacy studies of fluoxetine (Prozac) found that it was modestly effective in treating depression and resulted in response rates similar to those obtained in previous meta-analyses of tricyclic antidepressants (Greenberg et al 1994). Other meta-analyses and reviews have also found that new-generation antidepressants have equivalent outcomes to tricyclics (e.g. Anderson & Tomenson 1994, Edwards 1992, 1995, Kasper et al 1992).

It has been suggested that there may be some preference for SSRIs over tricyclics because they cause less sedation and fewer anticholinergic effects and cardiac complications than the standard tricyclics; however, they are associated with other side effects such as nausea, diarrhea, weight loss, agitation, anxiety, and insomnia (Edwards 1995; see Table 2.3 for details about the side effects of tricyclics, monoamine oxidase inhibitors (MAOIs), and SSRI antidepressants). Although drop-out rates from medication treatment studies are high regardless of the type of

TABLE 2.3	*Antidepressants, side effects, and mechanisms of action*		
Antidepressant type	**Generic names (Brand)**	**Side effects**	**Mechanism of action**
Monoamine oxidase inhibitors (MAOIs)	Phenelzine (Nardil) Tranylcypromine (Parnate)	The most serious side effect is a very rapid, very high, and dangerous increase in blood pressure caused by an interaction between the MAOI and foods containing tyramine. MAOIs interact with many other medications. Activating effects can interfere with sleep. Less common side effects include dry mouth, transient impotence, skin rash, and blurred vision	MAOIs block monoamine oxidase, which breaks down norepinephrine, serotonin, and dopamine. Therefore the functional levels of these neurotransmitters are increased

cont.

cont.

Antidepressant type	Generic names (Brand)	Side effects	Mechanism of action

Tricyclics (TCAs)	Tertiary TCAs
	  Amitriptyline (Elavil)
	  Clomipramine (Anafranil)
	  Doxepin (Sinequan)
	  Imipramine (Tofranil)
	  Trimipramine (Surmontil)
	Secondary TCAs
	  Desipramine (Norpramin)
	  Nortriptyline (Pamelor)
	  Protriptyline (Vivactil)
	  Amoxipine (Asendin)
	  Maprotiline (Ludiomil)
		Fatal when taken as an overdose. Potentiate the effect of alcohol. Dry mouth, blurred vision, constipation, heart palpitations, sweating, sedation. Cardiovascular side effects, weight gain, decreased libido and impotence. Like all antidepressants, tricyclics may trigger a manic episode in vulnerable individuals. May cause a decrease in blood pressure when the person stands	Tertiary TCAs are more potent blockers of serotonin reuptake, whereas secondary TCAs are more potent blockers of norepinephrine reuptake

Selective serotonin reuptake inhibitors (SSRIs)	Fluoxetine (Prozac) Fluvoxamine (Luvox) Paroxetine (Paxil) Sertraline (Zoloft)	Weight loss, activation rather than sedation, sometimes increased anxiety, nausea, and headaches. Sexual dysfunction. Benefits: less fatal after overdose than TCAs and fewer cardiac side effects	SSRIs selectively block the reuptake of serotonin into nerve cells in the brain
Atypical	Buproprion (Wellbutrin)	Agitation, insomnia, gastrointestinal upset, and headaches	Norepinephrine and serotonin are indirectly affected and dopamine reuptake is blocked
	Trazodone (Desyrel)	Priapism (painful, long-lasting erections) and dry mouth. Absence of anticholinergic effects	Potentiates serotonin
	Nefazodone (Serzone)	Nausea most common, dry mouth, dizziness	Related to trazodone but is less likely to cause priapism, and fewer cardiovascular effects
	Venlafaxine (Effexor)	Nausea, somnolence, dry mouth, dizziness, constipation, nervousness, sweating, and anorexia	Effexor blocks the reuptake of serotonin and norepinephrine without blocking other neurotransmitters
	Mirtazapine (Remeron)	Somnolence	Selectively blocks serotonin receptors

Sources: Diamond (1998), Keltner & Folks (1997), Maxmen & Ward (1995).

antidepressant used, the side effects of SSRIs may be slightly better tolerated by some people. These differences in tolerability are very small and may not be clinically meaningful. Furthermore, the number of patients completing each type of treatment is approximately equivalent (Greenberg & Fisher 1997).

The average effect in psychotherapy outcome research is one standard deviation, which is statistically large. An effect size of one standard deviation means that the average person receiving psychotherapy is better off than 84% of the people in the control condition who did not receive psychotherapy. In five meta-analyses of outcome with depression, psychotherapy outperformed no-treatment and wait-list controls (Lambert & Bergin 1994). Effect sizes produced by psychotherapy are equal to or greater than effects produced by various medical and educational interventions (Lambert & Bergin 1994).

For example, psychotherapy is as effective as or more effective than antidepressant medication (Dobson 1989, Robinson et al 1990, Steinbrueck et al 1983). When the allegiance of investigators and the differences between treatments are taken into account, the effectiveness of psychotherapy and pharmacotherapy is equivalent (Robinson et al 1990, Steinbrueck et al 1983). The results of the NIMH Collaborative Depression study, the largest and most well-controlled psychotherapy study conducted to date, support this notion. The NIMH study utilized investigators who were committed to each type of therapy compared and found little evidence for significant differences between therapies (Elkin et al 1989).

These findings are significant because antidepressants are often considered the treatment of choice for depression. Evans and colleagues (1992) found that psychotherapy may have an advantage over antidepressants in terms of decreased vulnerability to relapse. In addition, psychotherapy is not accompanied by the somatic side effects that occur with antidepressants. However, there is some evidence that antidepressants may start to work faster than psychotherapy and may be more effective with endogenous depressions (Lambert & Bergin 1994).

Relapse, Recurrence and the Role of Maintenance Treatments

Depression tends to be a chronic and recurrent disorder. A naturalistic study of depression found that 70% of people recover from depression after 1 year and 81% after 2 years. Unfortunately, 12% of depressed individuals do not recover until 5 years after the onset of the episode and 7% of individuals suffering from depression remain chronically depressed (Hirschfeld & Schatzberg 1994).

Even once successfully treated, depression is likely to recur. Without further treatment, one-fifth of previously recovered persons once again meet criteria for major depression 6 months after the completion of treatment, and nearly one-quarter will develop new depressive symptoms. Within 18 months, over one-third of those persons who were remitted will once again meet criteria for full depression (Shea et al 1992). Ten years after an initial episode, 76% of patients will have a recurrence of depression. For those who have experienced two episodes, there is an 80–90% chance of experiencing a third episode (Hirschfeld & Schatzberg 1994). A growing consensus among those who treat depression is that, after recovery, some form of continued maintenance treatment is necessary.

Whereas research into the pharmacotherapy of depression has provided ample data concerning response to acute treatment, much less is known about the long-term efficacy of antidepressants. The available data suggest that a substantial proportion (10–34%) of patients who have responded to pharmacotherapy experience a return of depression during continued treatment (Belsher & Costello 1988, Doogan & Caillard 1992, Evans et al 1992, Frank et al 1990, Montgomery et al 1988, Prien & Kupfer 1986, Prien et al 1984, Robinson et al 1991, Thase 1990). Even greater recurrence rates are reported during long-term treatment for more severe depression. For example, Prien et al (1984) reported a 52% recurrence rate in patients on imipramine and Glen (1984) reported 68–70% recurrence rate in those on amitriptyline or lithium. Taken together, these data highlight the recurrent nature of mood disorders even during the course of long-term treatment and magnify the importance of developing alternative approaches for both short- and long-term treatment of depression.

Only a few studies have examined the effectiveness of psychotherapy maintenance – continued treatment designed to help keep a person from returning to a depressed state. These studies indicate that maintenance psychotherapy (alone or in combination with pharmacotherapy) helps to prevent or delay relapse or recurrence of depression. Based on a limited number of studies, cognitive therapy appears to be an effective maintenance treatment and may delay the onset of subsequent episodes of depression (Blackburn et al 1986). Although following a 6-month continuation phase relapse rates did not differ between cognitive therapy, cognitive therapy plus antidepressant drug of choice (typically amitriptyline or clomipramine), and antidepressant-alone groups, those participants receiving cognitive therapy (alone and in combination with antidepressants) had a significantly lower relapse rate than patients receiving antidepressants alone. Even without maintenance, similar results were obtained in a 2-year follow-up (Evans et al 1992). At the end of a 2-year follow-up in which no maintenance treatments were provided, patients who had received cognitive therapy (with or without medication) had significantly lower relapse rates (21% and 15%) than those who had received antidepressants only (50%) during a 3-month acute treatment phase. Another group that was continued on antidepressants for the first year of follow-up had an intermediate relapse rate (32%), which did not differ significantly from that of the other groups. Limited sample sizes (10 to 13 per group), however, make interpretation of the nonsignificant difference precarious. Collectively, these findings suggest that cognitive therapy is at least as effective as antidepressant medication in preventing relapse or recurrence.

There are also indications that interpersonal psychotherapy (IPT) provides some benefit as a maintenance treatment. An 8-month maintenance study (Klerman et al 1974) found that weekly IPT produced lower relapse rates (17%) than placebo combined with monthly 15-min IPT sessions (31%). The group receiving IPT weekly performed almost as well as the groups receiving amitriptyline and monthly IPT (12% relapse) and the amitriptyline combined with weekly IPT group (12.5% relapse). A 3-year maintenance study (Frank et al 1990) found that IPT alone, given once a month, had a recurrence rate of 60%, a rate between that of the medication groups and the placebo group. It should be noted, however, that imipramine maintenance was given in a much higher dosage than in any previous maintenance study and IPT was given in a much lower dosage (monthly) than found effective in previous studies. Nonetheless, the IPT maintenance treatments significantly lengthened the mean time of remission (survival rate) to over 1 year, compared with the placebo group with a mean duration of remission of 38 weeks.

CAUSES OF DEPRESSION

Psychological Theories

Depression undoubtedly has many causes, and no single cause is likely to provide an adequate explanation. Different individuals may have different factors that contribute to their depression, and for any given individual multiple factors will contribute. Below we discuss some of the most widely researched factors that are thought to contribute to depression.

Learned Helplessness

The learned helplessness model posits that feelings of helplessness underlie depression. This model is based on research with both humans and animals, and has detailed how animals and humans learn that their efforts do not affect their situation and as a result they give up. Learning that behavior does not influence the situation causes motivational, cognitive, and emotional changes that resemble those in depression (Seligman 1975). Humans learn to feel helplessness not only by being in an uncontrollable situation, but also by coming to expect that their behavior will not affect important outcomes. When individuals stop expecting their responses to have an effect, they may cease trying. They have little motivation to try to escape or change situations because they have learned that nothing will change, despite their efforts. Learned helplessness also diminishes the chances that a person will later learn that responses do alter a situation. For example, dogs that were placed in a shuttle box and exposed to unavoidable inescapable shock later failed to attempt an escape when they were placed in a shuttle box in which they could escape the shock by jumping over the barrier. Learned helplessness produces affective deficits because an individual experiences negative cognitions as a result of learned helplessness (Abramson et al 1978).

The theory was revised when research demonstrated that most people do not become depressed when they experience an uncontrollable negative event. According to the reformulated theory (Abramson et al 1978), some people demonstrate a 'depressogenic' attributional style in which they explain negative events using internal, stable, and global reasons. Individuals can make either internal or external attributions about the reasons for negative events (e.g. it was my fault versus it was someone else's fault). Those who make internal attributions are likely to suffer a loss of self-esteem because they feel that the uncontrollable situation stems from their inadequacy, whereas those who make external attributions believe their helplessness is a result of the situation and realize that the situation will change (Abramson et al 1978).

Another factor that affects an individual's emotional reaction to an event is whether he or she generalizes the helplessness to all situations (makes a global attribution) or specifies that the helplessness occurs only in this particular situation (makes a specific attribution) (Abramson et al 1978). If individuals believe the negative event is due to a transitory factor (e.g. they failed the test because they did not feel well), they will make an unstable attribution that will result in only a short-lived depressive reaction. In contrast, a stable attribution about something that is unlikely to change will result in prolonged negative feelings about the event; for example, they failed the test because they are stupid (Abramson et al 1978). Research has demonstrated that an internal, stable, and global attributional style is a marker for vulnerability to depression (Seligman & Nolen-Hoeksema 1987).

Cognitive Model of Depression

According to the cognitive model of depression (Beck 1976), individuals become depressed because of inaccurate information processing that causes them to interpret events in a biased way. These negative but incorrect beliefs involve negative views of self, a negative world view, and pessimistic future expectations. These beliefs lead to behaviors that serve to reaffirm the beliefs. Furthermore, once they become depressed, individuals tend to focus selectively on negative thoughts, which cause them to perceive themselves and their situation in the worst possible light. This negative bias contributes to the maintenance of the depressed mood (Hollon & Garber 1988). Negative cognitions are viewed as necessary but not sufficient to trigger depression. They interact with other predisposing factors such as genetics, developmental factors, and traumatic events to trigger depression in certain individuals.

Gender Differences in Depression

The incidence of unipolar depression in women is approximately twice as high as the rate in men. According to Nolen-Hoeksema (1987), women tend to ruminate in response to depressed mood, amplifying and sustaining it, and men tend to cope with depressed mood by engaging in active behavior, which serves to inhibit their dysphoria. These differences in coping style may stem from social pressure on men to be active and ignore their moods, whereas women are socialized to be emotional and contemplative (Nolen-Hoeksema 1987).

Rumination contributes to depression by interfering with problem-solving behavior, which can lead to failure, feelings of helplessness, and exacerbation of the depressed mood. In contrast, active behavior can increase feelings of control, create reinforcement, and dampen depression. Furthermore, rumination increases an individual's focus on negative memories, and activates depressive explanations of the negative feelings, which in turn lead to decreased activity, increased chances of subsequent failure, and a perpetuation of feelings of depression and helplessness (Nolen-Hoeksema 1987).

Interpersonal Factors and Social Skills

Another factor believed to be important in buffering an individual from the effects of loss and other stressful life events is social support. Having few supportive social relationships, a small social network, and few close relationships are associated with increased depression. In addition, there is evidence to suggest that the supportiveness of the most intimate relationship plays the biggest role in buffering an individual from depression, and that other supportive relationships cannot make up for deficiencies in one's closest relationship (Coyne et al 1991).

Depression arises when negative life events lead to disappointment in expectations, personal goals, or plans. Marital discord is one example of such a stressor. Hammen (1991) has conducted longitudinal research in which she investigated individuals who were achievement focused and individuals who were socially focused. She found that individuals who experienced a life event that was considered a setback in the area of self-esteem focus were more likely to become depressed than those who experienced a setback in a domain that they were less invested in. One of the risk factors for depression is whether an individual experiences a negative life event that leads to a loss of self-esteem in an important area (e.g. an individual who derives most of her self-esteem from interpersonal relationships may become depressed when she experiences marital difficulties with her partner).

The negative life event may, in turn, cause the individual to experience reduced positive reinforcement and an increase in negative mood. The negative experience can trigger a negative self-focus that leads to self-criticism, unfavorable evaluations of one's own performance, blaming oneself for negative events, and negative expectations for the future.

There are behavioral consequences of self-focused attention, such as social withdrawal and interpersonal difficulties. Moreover, negative expectations may cause decreased effort and persistence on tasks. The overall effect of the self-esteem-damaging event can create conditions that perpetuate depression (Lewinsohn et al 1985).

Coping skills, such as the ability to see setback as opportunity (e.g. individuals who view losing their job as an opportunity to find a better job), can buffer the individual from loss of self-esteem. In addition, individuals who are able to decrease their self-focus by engaging in a distracting activity may be able to activate problem-solving skills rather than becoming caught up in rumination. Therefore, individuals who have predisposing characteristics (e.g. a confiding relationship or high learned resourcefulness) that permit them to cope effectively with a stressor will be able to stop the depressed feelings before they lead to a depressive episode, whereas those who lack these immunity factors or who have vulnerability factors may not be able to interrupt the depression feedback loop.

There is a complex interaction between predisposing characteristics and negative life events such that the presence of certain immunities may protect an individual from depression in spite of other vulnerability factors and, conversely, a particular combination of vulnerabilities may counteract the positive effect of an immunity factor. An individual's predisposing characteristics, both immunities and vulnerabilities to depression, mediate the reaction to stressful life events so that in some individuals these events lead to a disruption in expectations or plans and create depression, whereas other individuals can compensate for losses and interrupt the path to depression.

Biological Theories

Research suggests that both psychological and biological factors are important in contributing to the onset of depression. People who are depressed often show signs of dysregulation of circadian rhythms (e.g. greater depression at certain times of the day), sleep disturbance, and alteration of eating habits. Psychological events can trigger this dysregulation and the depression that follows may be accompanied by altered psychological thought processes as well as maladaptive biological changes (Shelton et al 1991). It can be challenging, however, to establish whether depression is linked to a particular event. Even when there is a precipitating event, this can change as the depression continues. There are frequently clear triggers for an initial episode of major depression but not for later episodes (Brown et al 1994). Currently there is no solid evidence that certain types of depression are caused 'biologically' and others 'psychologically', and there is some evidence to the contrary (Rush & Weissenburger 1994). There is, however, evidence that treatments that alter biological rhythms, such as sleep deprivation, decreasing time spent in rapid eye movement (REM) sleep, and receiving light therapy, can relieve symptoms in many depressed individuals (Shelton et al 1991). These findings led to the development of the dysregulation hypothesis of depression.

Depression as Dysregulation

Individuals have 'zeitgebers' (time-givers): personal relationships, social demands, and behaviors that keep biological rhythms regulated normally. For example, one has to wake up at a certain time to go to work. Ehlers et al (1988) believe that these social interactions are the important link between psychological and biological aspects of depression. If a person loses social reinforcement – perhaps through death of a loved one or loss of a job – there is a resulting dysregulation of biological rhythms resulting in symptoms (e.g. mood disturbance, sleep disturbance, eating disturbance, psychomotor changes, and fatigue) that we call depression. In addition, treatments that reset the 'biological clock' are effective in alleviating depression in many individuals. Moreover, there are high rates of depression in people who work swing shift or night shift, who are more likely to experience disturbances in their biological rhythms.

Genetics

There is a hereditary component contributing to the predisposition to develop a mood disorder. Family studies demonstrate that first-degree relatives of those with major depressive disorder are 1.5–3 times more likely to develop depression than the general population. The risk for first-degree relatives of patients with bipolar disorder is 10 times the risk for the general population (Strober et al 1988).

Twin studies indicate that bipolar disorder is more heritable than major depressive disorder. In addition, the fact that there is a higher concordance rate between monozygotic (identical) twins than between dizygotic (fraternal) twins for major depression (40% versus 11%) and bipolar disorder (72% versus 14%) supports the heritability of depression in general (Allen 1976). An adoption study conducted by Mendlewicz & Ranier (1977) found that 31% of biological parents of bipolar adoptees had mood disorders, compared with 2% of the biological parents of normal adoptees. Another study (Wender et al 1986) found that biological relatives of those with a broad range of mood disorders were eight times more likely to have major depression than biological relatives of individuals who were not diagnosed with any mood disorders.

Neurotransmitter Function

It has been hypothesized that abnormal levels of, or function of, neurotransmitters such as norepinephrine (NE), dopamine, and serotonin are a possible cause of depression. It was originally believed that decreased levels of NE contributed to the development of depressive symptoms. This is unlikely to be the mechanism, however, because most antidepressant medications take several weeks to have an impact on depression, but they have an immediate effect on blocking the reuptake of NE and other neurotransmitters. Research suggests that antidepressants may work by increasing the sensitivity of the postsynaptic receptors for NE, which appear to be undersensitive in depressed individuals (Siever & Davis 1985). Furthermore, research indicates that serotonin dysregulation is also involved in the onset of depression. L-Tryptophan, an amino acid involved in the synthesis of serotonin, is an effective treatment for both mania and depression (Prange et al 1974). Prange and colleagues have proposed a combined norepinephrine–serotonin hypothesis which states that: (1) a serotonin deficiency increases vulnerability to mood disorder, and (2) when there is a serotonin deficiency, too much NE will result in mania, and too little NE will trigger depression (Prange et al 1974).

TREATMENTS FOR DEPRESSION

Psychological Treatments

The most widely used treatments for depression include psychotherapy and antidepressant treatment. Until recently, antidepressants were considered to be a more effective treatment than psychotherapy. Psychotherapy, however, appears to produce outcomes equivalent to those obtained with antidepressants (Elkin et al 1989), and with fewer side effects. In addition, there is some evidence that psychotherapy may protect against or delay relapsing after treatment has stopped (Evans et al 1992).

When choosing a treatment for a patient, it is important to keep in mind his or her preferences and personality characteristics. Individuals are more likely to respond to a preferred treatment because they believe that it will work, and are less likely to discontinue the treatment. Certain individuals may be more likely to respond to one or another treatment, although the current state of knowledge does not assist in selecting the most effective treatment on the basis of assessing patient characteristics.

Interpersonal Psychotherapy

IPT is directed towards helping individuals interact more effectively with others. It focuses on the individual's history of maladaptive behaviors that have created negative interactions, and seeks to alter those behaviors, thoughts, and feelings in order to result in more positive relationships. It also looks for links in the present behavior to past experiences in childhood that may have caused the patient to learn those ineffective social skills. Together, the patient and therapist explore the problems and attempt to alter the behavior and consequently relationships over time (Ehlers et al 1988). Research suggests that IPT is an effective treatment for depression and is as effective as antidepressant treatment and other forms of psychotherapy (Elkin et al 1989).

Cognitive Therapy

Cognitive therapy aims to change patients' maladaptive belief systems to create more acceptable reactions to people and healthier interpretations of situations (Ehlers et al 1988). The patient and therapist explore the patient's negative beliefs and the patient engages in hypothesis-testing activities to disconfirm his or her erroneous views (Hollon & Garber 1988).

The patient and therapist engage in a dialogue to define the problem, help the patient identify his or her assumptions, determine the importance of events to the patient, and point out the disadvantages of retaining the biased beliefs and maladaptive behaviors. The patient develops new skills that teach him or her to alter negative thoughts and become more independent (Corsini & Wedding 1989).

The main goal of cognitive therapy is to teach patients to alter their faulty information processing so that they interpret events in an adaptive way. The therapist aims to help patients develop new skills which they can use to prevent a recurrence of the depression. In final sessions the patients are asked to imagine themselves in difficult situations and decide what they would do if such an instance arose (Hollon & Garber 1988). Research suggests that cognitive therapy is as effective as antidepressant treatment and other forms of psychotherapy in treating depression (Elkin et al 1989).

Biological Treatments

Antidepressant Treatment

Tricyclic medications are commonly used to treat depression (e.g. imipramine and amitriptyline). The mechanism of tricyclic agents is to block the reuptake of neurotransmitters (especially NE and dopamine) from the space between the neurons in the brain (synaptic cleft). Numerous controlled double-blind research studies have demonstrated that tricyclics have efficacy in the treatment of depression (Goodwin 1992). Like most antidepressant medications, tricyclics take approximately 2–3 weeks to affect the depression (Delgado et al 1992).

Monoamine oxidase inhibitor (MAOI) antidepressants began to be used about the same time as tricyclics, but they are not as widely used. MAOIs may cause high blood pressure when used in conjunction with foods that contain tyramine (e.g. cheese and chocolate). Some early research indicated that they are not as effective as tricyclics; however, a recent review concluded that when used with a proper diet they are an effective treatment for depression (Larsen 1991).

Selective serotonin reuptake inhibitors (SSRIs; e.g. Prozac and Zoloft) are a relatively new class of drugs synthesized in the early 1980s. They work by blocking the reuptake of serotonin so that increased levels remain in the synaptic cleft. They have a high selectivity for blocking serotonin reuptake receptors, whereas tricyclics affect to a greater extent both NE and other neurotransmitters. SSRIs are currently the most frequently prescribed medication. Controlled trials suggest that they are equivalent in effectiveness to the tricyclics; however, they have fewer side effects, are more easily adjusted to the proper dosage level, and are less toxic if the patient overdoses (Greenberg & Fisher 1997). Table 2.3 summarizes each type of medication, side effects, and mechanism of action.

Electroconvulsive Therapy (ECT)

ECT is usually administered to inpatients in a series of treatments. Treatment frequency is approximately twice a week. Many people demonstrate marked improvement after six to eight sessions, but some need more. Electrodes are placed either on both sides of the head or at the front and back of the skull on one side of the head. ECT remains an effective treatment according to several studies (Consensus Conference 1985), although the mechanism through which it works is still unknown (Sackheim 1989). ECT is usually reserved for severely depressed patients who have not responded to other forms of treatment or who are at immediate risk of suicide. ECT may also be more effective than medication with rapid cycling bipolar patients and depressed patients with psychotic symptoms. Although infrequent, ECT can result in pervasive and persistent memory loss. More frequently, it results in minor memory loss for events that happen shortly before receiving treatment, but does not result in persistent memory loss.

MULTIPLE TREATMENT APPROACHES AND ETIOLOGIES

Some clinicians believe that certain types of depression have a biological etiology and others have a psychological etiology. The literature suggests, however, that there are a number of different possible causes of depression, each involving a complex interaction between biological, psychological, and social factors. No one perspective provides a complete explanation for how depression develops. Regardless of how the episode appears to be precipitated, the causal mechanisms are affected at all three levels: biological, psychological, and social. While medications seem to intervene at a biological level and psychotherapy treats depression at a psychosocial level, both interrupt the chain of events that maintains the depression and both facilitate changes in the other domains. For example, antidepressants affect neurotransmitter receptor sensitivity but also affect how individuals interact with others once they begin to feel better. Psychotherapy initially targets behavior change or cognitive change (e.g. socializing with others or learning not to make minor setbacks into devastating events), which then triggers physiological changes as well.

It is important to remember that the cause of depression cannot be explained with a simple biological or psychological explanation alone. The likelihood that any given individual becomes depressed is the result of a complex interaction of heredity, physiology, environmental events, cognitive representations, and situational factors. Treatment can intervene at any point in this complex web and have effects on function across all arenas. In this early stage of research into the effectiveness of acupuncture, it is important to keep in mind that the impact of acupuncture may be seen in physiological, psychological, and social domains, but that such effects do not address the ultimate question of precisely how acupuncture works in the treatment of depression.

3 | Chinese Medicine Theory

INTRODUCTION

Although any acupuncturist using this manual would be knowledgeable of the basic concepts of Chinese Medicine (CM), and would probably be familiar with the eight guiding criteria as a style of treatment, a complete section on the theoretical framework is included. This has been done for the sake of continuity as well as to introduce the nonacupuncture community to the Chinese Medicine conceptualization of depression. The aim is not only to provide a clinical tool for acupuncture practitioners but also to foster understanding and collaboration between acupuncturists, psychotherapists, physicians, and researchers.

Theoretical References

In the development of our treatment protocol for depression, we sought to integrate five areas or 'filters' (Seem 1985) which serve as the basis for assessment and treatment in acupuncture:

1. Yin/yang and eight guiding criteria
2. Viscera and bowels

3. Qi, blood and body fluids
4. Channels and network vessels
5. Five phases.

The pilot study outlined in Chapter 7, as well the framework for this manual, are based primarily on the first three filters: (1) the eight guiding criteria, (2) viscera and bowels, and (3) qi, blood, and body fluids. These three filters are generally used together as a unit. Although the different theories that serve as the foundation for the five areas can be artificially compartmentalized, in reality they function together as a whole, and are all necessary to understand the etiology and progression of imbalances. The approach presented in this manual aims to integrate what we have found to be the most useful features of each 'filter' in the evaluation and treatment of depression, while emphasizing the use of the eight guiding criteria, viscera and bowels, and qi, blood and body fluids, as the foundation for treatment design. All five areas mentioned above are used in some way to explain the disease mechanisms that underlie depression, to understand the pattern differentiation characteristic of depressive episodes, and to outline the treatment principles and treatment strategies for point selection. We use the step-by-step methodology characteristic of eight principles pattern identification: (1) differentiate signs and symptoms using the four evaluations, (2) establish disease mechanisms, patterns, and pattern combinations, (3) outline treatment principles, and (4) design a treatment plan. We have, however, deviated from what is commonly known as traditional Chinese Medicine (TCM) in essentially three ways: first, we make extensive use of the five-phase theory in the initial interview to determine the specific nature of each person's experience of depression; second, we encourage palpation of the abdominal area, and the channels for point selection; and third, we modify our point selection and total strategy over time, on the basis of channel interactions that are not emphasized in TCM. Such channel interactions are more broadly used by the Vietnamese and French acupuncture schools, some Japanese acupuncture styles, and the acupuncture style developed by Dr Mark Seem.[1]

After having used this manual extensively, as both a clinical and a teaching tool, it became obvious that the treatment strategies that had been used consistently as part of our treatment protocol expanded the framework beyond the TCM model. The rationale for point selection, point combinations, and point location, although based on TCM

---

[1]TCM is a style of Chinese Medicine that emerged predominantly from the People's Republic of China in the twentieth century, and which is presented as the standard model of Chinese Medicine in mainland China today. For an interesting discussion of TCM, its history, development, and clinical standards, see Fruehauf (1999).

pattern differentiation, was heavily influenced by training under Mark Seem. Seem's approach developed through the influence of the French energetic school of acupuncture, and the work of Dr Van Ghi. For this reason, the section that describes the channels and network vessels deviates from standard TCM theory to include a broader consideration of the complexity of the channel system, which has very little importance in TCM as a style of treatment today. Although purists in any of these traditions may argue against combining different styles of treatment, in reality the contemporary practice of acupuncture has emerged as a 'weaving of lineages within the diverse traditions that make up Oriental medicine' (Hougham 2000). In line with this view, the authors hope to make a small contribution towards the development of a foundation for a multidimensional energetic approach to the assessment and treatment of depression – one that allows the practitioner to stratify treatment options based on an integrated use of the five filters. It needs to be emphasized, however, that any system that may emerge from this endeavor – to be authentic and internally coherent – must develop on a solid foundation: one that is based on a clearly articulated theoretical framework and a consistent treatment methodology.

The authors recognize the validity and significance of diverse schools of thought in the treatment of depression with acupuncture. We selected the eight guiding criteria as the primary framework for our study because in our view: (1) the eight criteria offer a methodological approach that can be more easily replicated in control studies, (2) most of the existing research literature for acupuncture in the treatment of depression uses the eight guiding criteria directly or indirectly, (3) the reference literature available in English is based on these criteria, and (4) the eight guiding criteria as a style of treatment offers more consistent treatment protocols. It is of great interest to the authors to be able to compare – in the future – different styles of treatment and their clinical outcomes, but this was not an aim of our pilot study, nor of this book.

In order to establish a parallel between Western-defined major depression and acupuncture patterns of disharmony, we looked at depression as a complex interplay of disease mechanisms that develop from three main factors: (1) the patient's predisposing tendency towards vacuity or repletion of either yin or yang, (2) the liver's inability to maintain the free and smooth flow of qi, and (3) a disturbance in the heart's function of housing the spirit (*shen*). In Table 3.1, for the sake of convenience, the clinical symptoms of depression are grouped under the four headings described in Box 3.1.

In this way, the question we pose within the context of Chinese Medicine is not only whether someone is depressed, but *how* this

TABLE 3.1	A comparison of the symptoms of Western-defined depression and patterns of disharmony defined by Chinese medicine			
DSM-IV symptoms	**Yin features**[a]	**Yang features**[b]	**Qi stagnation**	**Shen disturbance**
Depressed mood	Depressed mood with lethargy and weakness, lower libido, decreased motivation	Depressed mood with irritability, uneasiness, anxiety, violent outbursts of anger, aggression	Depressed mood with emotional liability, periodic outbursts of anger, frustration, erratic physical complaints, migratory pains, distension of breast and abdomen, sighing	Depressed mood characterized by flat affect
Diminished interest or pleasure	Diminished interest or pleasure			Diminished interest or pleasure
Fatigue or loss of energy	Fatigue or loss of energy			
Appetite disturbance	Appetite disturbance characterized by loss of appetite with weak digestion; tendency towards loose stools or diarrhea	Appetite disturbance characterized by excessive appetite, bitter taste in the mouth, thirst	Appetite disturbance characterized by indigestion with belching, nausea, bloating, flatulence, belching. Erratic elimination	
Sleep disturbance	Hypersomnia	Dream-disturbed sleep; nightmares		Insomnia with difficulty falling or staying asleep, or waking up early
Psychomotor agitation or retardation	Decreased energy level, slow body movements, no desire to move or talk	Inability to sit still, pacing, agitation, nervousness, wiriness		Incessant, nervous talking. Slow, soft, monotonous speech; muteness or decreased speech; increased pauses
Worthlessness; excessive or inappropriate guilt	Excessive or inappropriate guilt		Both features when accompanied by frustration and periodic outbursts of anger	Feelings of worthlessness
Diminished ability to think or concentrate; indecisiveness	Both features when accompanied by apathy and lethargy	Both features when accompanied by agitation and restlessness	Indecisiveness when accompanied by frustration	Diminished ability to think or concentrate
Recurrent thoughts of death, suicidal ideation or attempt	Recurrent suicidal ideation, no plans and no attempts	Recurrent suicidal ideation, possibly more attempts	Recurrent suicidal ideation with a specific plan	Recurrent suicidal ideation with or without a plan
Other symptoms or associated features	Brooding or rumination. Phobias. Excessive concern with physical symptoms	Anxiety, panic attacks, phobias	Tearfulness, irritability, excessive concern with physical health. Panic attacks with agoraphobia	Tearfulness, anxiety, panic attacks

[a] Tendency towards vacuity of qi or yang with possible yin repletion.
[b] Tendency towards vacuity of yin with possible yang repletion.

BOX 3.1	*Chinese Medicine grouping of the clinical symptoms of depression*

Yin features Symptoms that are primarily yin in nature and which manifest as either a tendency towards qi and yang *vacuity* (yang), and/or *repletion* of dampness and phlegm (yin).

Yang features Symptoms that are primarily yang in nature and which manifest as either a tendency towards yin and blood *vacuity* (yin) and/or *repletion* of heat or fire (yang).

Qi stagnation Symptoms that develop from the liver's inability to perform its function of coursing and discharge.

Shen disturbance Symptoms that develop from either *vacuity* or *repletion* patterns which affect the heart's ability to house the spirit (*shen*).

person is experiencing depression, and what precipitating factors – physical, psychological, and social – have contributed to his or her present condition. Chinese Medicine offers, then, a framework for understanding distinct symptom pictures and for developing a treatment approach based on the nature of *each individual's* particular symptom pattern. Thus acupuncture treatments focus on the entire symptom picture, which includes physiological as well as psychiatric symptoms.

THE ASSESSMENT OF DEPRESSION WITHIN THE FRAMEWORK OF TRADITIONAL CHINESE MEDICINE

Chinese philosophy is based on the premise that all life occurs within a unified system, that all phenomena are manifestations of a unifying principle of energy or life force, and that all manifestations of life are connected and mutually dependent upon one another. Life unfolds as a process of differentiation that expresses the interaction between two complementary forces, yin and yang, which represent the totality of the dynamic equilibrium. This unified system is understood as a process of fluctuations and permanent change, as the cyclic nature of continuous movement. Everything can be characterized as either yin or yang, relative aspects of an alternating cycle along a single continuum (Beinfield & Korngold 1991). The creative principle that symbolizes life in all its forms and which activates every process that characterizes living entities is known as qi (pronounced 'chee') or 'vital energy', and is central to Chinese medical theory.

Human beings are considered a microcosm that reflects the universe that surrounds them – a dynamic series of energetic fluctuations constitutes the body as a living system (Seem 1987). Each of us is an ecosystem living within a larger ecosystem. The balance of forces within us determines our health and disease (Beinfield & Korngold 1991).

Acupuncture looks for disharmonies of qi and, strictly speaking, depression does not exist as a disease category in Chinese Medicine. When an acupuncturist using the eight-principles framework is asked to evaluate a 'depressed' person, he or she weaves all relevant information into a *pattern of disharmony*, a description of the dynamics that portray a situation of an imbalance. Symptoms are part of this imbalance which can be seen in other aspects of the patient's life and behavior (Kaptchuck 1983). Because the patient is always considered as a body–mind continuum, somatic and psychological symptoms are equally important.

By focusing on the detection of qi imbalances, rather than on the diagnosis and treatment of disease, Chinese Medicine explains relationships between physiological and psychological events that are considered separate phenomena in the Western medical model. Chinese Medicine offers a physiology that postulates a clear connection between somatic events and psychological concepts of mind and emotion, helping to close the gap between soma and psyche (Seem 1987). As with any other diagnostic system, the theoretical framework provided by Chinese Medicine can be used to understand the appearance of symptoms that characterize depression, to account for the heterogeneity of symptom presentation in depression, and to devise individually-tailored treatments for particular constellations of depressive symptoms.

CHINESE MEDICINE CONCEPTS OF ILLNESS AND HEALTH

Chinese Medicine defines health as the balance between yin and yang, which depends on the capacity of an organism to adapt to change and maintain equilibrium. Sickness is the result of vacuity or repletion of either yin or yang. *Vacuity* is defined as: weakness of the forces (right qi) that maintain the health of the body and fight disease, an insufficiency of vital substances (yin, blood, body fluids, essence; i.e. yin humor), or the diminished capacity of physiological processes. *Repletion* is defined as: an accumulation of physiological products (phlegm, dampness, blood, and qi) that are harmful to the body and may obstruct functioning, or as the relative excess of either endogenous or exogenous pathogens[2] that may threaten the health of

[2]In Chinese Medicine endogenous or exogenous pathogens are known as 'evil qi' (*xie*). They include the six qi (wind, cold, fire, summerheat, dampness, and dryness) in their capacity to cause disease; the 'warm evils' (warm heat school), and various types of toxins. Additional pathogens are *wind, cold, fire, dampness and dryness* arising within the body, and static blood and phlegm produced by the body (Wiseman & Feng 1998).

the organism. Vacuity and repletion are both imbalances between yin and yang.

The homeostasis of an organism – the balance between yin and yang – is sustained by the proper circulation of qi along energetic pathways or meridians, commonly known as the *channels* and *network vessels*. The channels form a network that connects the surface of the body with the internal organs (viscera and bowels), serving as a two-way communication system, which both conveys messages to the surface about internal malfunctioning and alerts the internal functions about surface phenomena that might be threatening to move deeper into the system (Seem 1987). The channels and network vessels are the surface manifestations of the viscera and bowels, and act as an irrigation system that regulates the supply of qi and prevents accumulations. The internal organs in Chinese Medicine are defined by their functions and interrelations, rather than by their somatic structures or specific anatomic locations. They work as spheres of influence, and represent a complete set of functions that reflect energetic relationships among physiological and psychological events. In order not to confuse them with the biomedical entities of the same name, we refer to them as *viscera* (yin) and *bowels* (yang); they are also sometimes referred to as organic–energetic functional units, organ functions (Seem 1987), organ networks (Beinfield & Korngold 1991), or energetic orbs (Porkert 1983). There are five viscera and six bowels. The viscera and bowels and the channels both work in pairs, with one yin and one yang function interconnected:[3] lung–large intestine, stomach–spleen, heart–small intestine, kidney–bladder, pericardium–triple heater, liver–gall bladder, yin and yang respectively.

In the sections that follow some of the basic concepts that serve as a foundation for Chinese medical treatment of depression are defined.

Yin and Yang

The Chinese characters for yin and yang denote the sunny and shady sides of a mountain respectively. These two complementary and opposing principles are used to describe phenomena that have a similar quality and relationship, including the different functions and

---

[3]The pericardium is considered as an extension of the functions of the heart and it is said to act as a buffer that protects the heart from external influences; it is not considered a separate viscera. In the context of the channels and network vessels, the pericardium is a channel in its own right and is considered the yin pair of the triple heater channel. Therefore, there are five (yin) viscera and six (yang) bowels; but there are six yin and six yang channels or meridians.

BOX 3.2	*Yin–yang correspondences*

Yin	**Yang**
Interior	Exterior
Weakness, depletion (vacuity)	Strength, fullness (repletion)
Cold	Heat
Blood	Qi
Viscera	Bowels
Lower, frontal, right parts of the body	Upper, dorsal, left parts of the body
Darkness, night, moon	Light, day, sun
Winter, midnight	Summer, midday
Heavy, dense, hard	Light, porous, soft
Form, substance, potential	Function, movement, action
Eco-active, sensible, aware of surroundings	Ego-centered, aggressive, aware of itself
Receptive, responsive, introverted, quiet	Demanding, extroverted, expressive

parts of the body. Yin and yang are rooted in each other: they are interdependent, relative to one another, divisible but inseparable. Yin and Yang counterbalance and complement each other and transform into each other (Box 3.2).

The potential for differentiation into yin and yang (*earlier heaven*), upon which life depends, is received from our parents at conception and stored in the kidney. The kidney has a very special relationship with the other viscera and bowels because it holds the foundation for their own yin and yang (Kaptchuk 1983). Each of the other viscera and bowels is considered to have a yin (storing, nourishing, cooling) component and a yang (activating, protective, warming) component, which are said to stem from the yin and yang roots of the kidney, respectively (Seem 1987). According to Kaptchuk (1983), yin is what sustains and conserves the organism and grants us the qualities of rest, tranquility, and quiescence; yin condenses and concentrates inwardly the energy of life. Yin moistens, softens, stabilizes, and roots life, and grants us the capacity to unfold gracefully while being content, quiet, and present. When yin is insufficient, we lack the qualities of receptivity and contemplation and become easily agitated, unsettled or nervously uneasy; the control over the dynamic manifestations of heat and activity is lost (Kaptchuk 1987). Yin represents the latent potential that awaits to be expressed and organized (Seem 1987).

Yang, by contrast, causes transformation and change, providing us with the capacity to engage life, to react, and to respond. Yang expands and disperses outwardly, granting the basic animating and invigorating quality of life that expresses our capacity to move, activate, and transform. When yang is insufficient, we find ourselves paralyzed in fear, confused and indecisive, unable to express what we want, hopeless. When the quickening power to move is lost, the expression of life becomes soggy, congested, inactive, and frozen (Kaptchuk 1987).

Usually, we can detect in every person a relative vacuity of either the yin or yang roots of the kidney, which will affect in turn the relative vacuity or repletion (hypoactivity or hyperactivity) of the associated yin or yang viscera and bowels (Seem 1987). These tendencies, which can be both trait and circumstantial, will influence the manner in which an individual responds to his or her environment and the stressors therein.

When considering the human being as a smaller system living within a larger system, individuals' relationships to their environment become of the utmost importance in the development of illness. Each of us will experience an event and react to a stressor in a different way. Our predisposition to develop a disorder at any given time depends on our individual experience of being in the world. Situations that create a conflict between our internal needs and desires and the demands placed upon us precipitate personal patterns of reaction based on our relative vacuity or repletion of either yin or yang (Seem 1987).

Based on this model, major depression can be considered as a 'somatic energetic reaction pattern' that is fueled by psychological and physical energies that are unique to the individual and that affect the experience of the disorder and nature of the symptoms. Moreover, this somatic energetic reaction pattern will influence the treatment protocol and prognosis. Stated differently, although persons with major depression may share common symptoms, for each individual the dynamics of dysfunction would have developed in such a way that will require individualized treatment based on differential energetic diagnosis.

Fundamental Substances: Qi, Blood, Essence, Spirit, and Body Fluids

Qi

Qi is the capacity of life to maintain and transform itself (Kaptchuk 1989). Qi has its own movement and activates the movement of other things; all physical and mental activities are manifestations of qi, and qi is perceived functionally by what it does (Beinfield & Korngold 1991). Sometimes referred to as 'vital energy' or simply 'energy', the concept of qi is much broader: qi is what motivates all movement, transformation, and change. According to Chinese Medicine, qi has five functions: defense, transformation, warming, restraint, and transportation. Qi protects the exterior of the body from invasion by external pathogens; it transforms substances so that they can be used by the organism; it provides warmth for the entire body; it holds the organs and substances in their proper place; and it propels all movement and transportation in the body.

Blood

According to Chinese Medicine blood is the substance that nourishes and moistens our body tissues. Blood is derived from food by the stomach and spleen, it is governed by the heart, stored in the liver, and moved through the vessels by the combined action of the heart and lung. When the blood is scanty or insufficient, no functions can take place; the blood moistens all body tissues, including the ligaments and tendons known as *sinews* in Chinese Medicine, as well as the skin and the eyes. Without proper nourishment and moisture, the tissues of the body can stiffen, dry out, and wither.

Blood and qi are very closely interrelated. In the human body, qi is the yang in relation to blood, which is the yin. The qi moves the blood, and the blood provides the material foundation for the qi. Blood, being yin in nature, provides *nourishment* and *moistening*, as well as the *material foundation* for the *shen* or spirit, which is yang. By accumulating in the heart, the blood helps to house and anchor the *shen*, and keep it rooted in the body (Schnyer & Flaws 1998). Later on, we will look in detail at some of the mental and emotional symptoms experienced during depressive episodes, which result from insufficiency or stagnation of blood.

Spirit

The Chinese concept of *shen*, or spirit, corresponds to the mental capacity to think, feel, and respond; it is what allows us to be conscious and alert during the day, and what becomes inactive during sleep. In that sense, *shen* refers to the Western concept of 'mind' (Wiseman & Feng 1998). In Chinese Medicine *shen* represents the accumulation of qi and blood in the heart; sufficient qi and blood accumulating in the heart are necessary to give rise to consciousness or spirit (Schnyer & Flaws 1998). Because *shen* is considered to have a material basis, its importance in medicine is not independent of the body. Kaptchuk (1983) refers to *shen* as the capacity of the mind to form ideas and the desire of the personality to live life. Human consciousness, memory, mental and emotional faculties, and awareness all indicate the presence of *shen*. For there to be consciousness and awareness, there needs to be sufficient qi; for the spirit to be quiet and calm, there needs to be enough blood to nourish it and settle it. Without sufficient blood (yin), the *shen* or spirit (yang) becomes restless; without enough qi our mental clarity is impeded (Schnyer & Flaws 1998).

Essence

Essence is the most fundamental, essential material the body utilizes for its growth, maturation, and reproduction (Schnyer & Flaws 1998). Essence determines the strength of the constitution. In women, the outward manifestation of essence is blood; in men it is semen. There are two forms of this essence: *inherited essence*, which is the constitutional basis acquired from our parents, and *acquired essence*, derived from the food and liquids we consume and the air we breathe. The natural process of living is the way in which we utilize this essence; we come to the world with a limited supply of inherited essence, our lifestyle choices determine the rate with which we use up this supply. Because all body functions depend on this essence, and because inherited essence cannot be replaced, it is very important to conserve it.

According to Chinese Medicine our inherited essence is a reservoir, and it is the acquired essence we create by eating, drinking, and breathing that provides the foundation for the qi and blood we utilize for our daily activities. If we eat properly, and through digestion we transform food and drink efficiently into nourishment (qi and blood), we produce sufficient qi and blood to perform our day-to-day activities. If, in addition, we have a good night's sleep, any surplus of qi and blood that was not utilized during the day goes on to bolster our inherited essence and become part of our reservoir (Schnyer & Flaws 1998). Inherited essence is governed and stored by the kidney; acquired essence is governed by the spleen.

This is, in part, the reason why digestion and diet are instrumental in understanding the mechanisms that underlie chronic and recurrent depression, why depression is more prevalent in women than in men (Kessler et al 1994), and why aging may be a risk factor in depression (Beekman et al 1999).

Body Fluids

The concept of body fluids comprises all the normal fluid substances of the human body; this term refers to fluids actually flowing within the human body, and to sweat, saliva, stomach juices, urine, and other fluids secreted or discharged by the body (Wiseman & Feng 1998). The body fluids are therefore different to the previous four concepts, as these fluids are the same as would be described in Western medicine. Body fluids in Chinese Medicine are differentiated as *liquid* fluids, which are thinner, mobile, and relatively yang in quality, and *humor*, which are thicker, less mobile, more turbid, yin fluids. The main function of the fluids is to keep the viscera and bowels, the skin, the hair, and the body orifices moistened; additionally, they lubricate the joints and nourish the brain, marrow and bones (Wiseman & Feng 1998).

The formation, distribution, and discharge of fluids involve complex processes in which several viscera and bowels play important roles. The processing of fluids begins in the stomach, where the useful part of the fluids (*essential qi*) is absorbed. The spleen carries this essential qi to the lungs, from where it is distributed to the other parts of the body. The small intestine separates the clear from the turbid, whereas the large intestine further absorbs fluid while conveying the waste material downward. Finally, the kidney plays the most important role in the formation and replacement of fluids by providing the warming and activating force for the other viscera and bowels to perform their roles; in addition, the kidney is responsible for transforming the surplus and waste fluid into urine, to be later discharged by the bladder.

VISCERA AND BOWELS

The relationship between the concepts of viscera and bowels in Chinese Medicine and the organs as we know them in Western medicine is mostly of name and not of function. As mentioned above, the organs of Chinese Medicine represent a complete set of functions, both psychological and physiological, and are defined by their interaction rather than by their anatomic structure. Each viscus and bowel has a responsibility for maintaining the physical and mental health of the organism. The viscera (relatively yin organs) store the essence and are responsible for creating and transforming qi and blood; the bowels (relatively yang organs) decompose food and convey waste. As mentioned above, there are five viscera – liver, heart, spleen, lung, and kidney (the pericardium is considered a sixth viscus in channel theory) – and six bowels: gall bladder, small intestine, stomach, large intestine, urinary bladder, and triple heater. The viscera and bowels are paired by functional relationship, respectively.

Liver

> 'The Liver holds the office of General of the armed forces. Assessment of circumstances and conception of plans stem from it.' (Su Wen, Ch. 8; cited in Larre & Rochat de la Vallée 1985, p. 34)

The liver controls 'coursing and discharge', meaning that it regulates the smooth and unobstructed flow of qi and blood. The liver maintains the uninhibited and free movement of qi throughout the body in order to prevent stagnation.

According to Hammer (1990), the liver is the first line of emotional defense for the entire organism; when confronted by a noxious emotional stimulus, this energy system is the organism's first choice for coping with the stressor. The liver deals with the stressors by assuring constant movement and circulation of qi, thus preventing stagnation.

The liver network expresses the capacity for growth, development, expression and change. Any experience that would inhibit this potential would directly affect the ability of the liver to maintain free flow. Any intense emotion that would find no release through verbal expression or physical activity would increase the demand on the nervous system for qi and blood, and would potentially render the liver incapable of renewing and circulating noxious energy (Hammer 1990). A condition of blockage or stagnation of qi would set in. Emotions, and especially anger and frustration, are the primary causes of liver qi stagnation.

Liver qi stagnation affects, in turn, other functions of the liver such as storing the blood and regulating digestion. It may also manifest as a blockage along the pathway of the liver channel (which traverses the pelvis, abdomen, chest, throat, gingiva, and head). Depending on the viability of the organ systems in a particular individual, liver depression qi stagnation[4] may affect the functions of other viscera and bowels. The combination of liver depression with predisposing factors precipitates, in turn, the cascade of disease mechanisms that characterizes each distinct pattern of disharmony present during depression. We will explain further the concept of qi stagnation, its relationship to depression, its complications and ramifications.

Because the first effect of the emotions as causative factors of disease is to upset the liver's function of coursing and discharge (i.e. the movement and transformation of qi and its proper circulation and direction), liver depression qi stagnation is likely to always be a significant factor in mental–emotional problems.

---

[4]The term 'liver depression qi stagnation' is a technical one used in Chinese Medicine to denote a particular disease mechanism and pattern of disharmony that involves the liver and that implies qi stagnation due to emotional stress and frustration (Wiseman & Feng 1998).

Heart

> 'The Heart holds the office of Lord and Sovereign. The radiance of the spirits stems from it.' (Su Wen, Ch. 8; cited in Larre & Rochat de la Vallée 1985, p. 23)

The heart is considered to be the emperor of the bodymind, the governor of the five viscera and the six bowels. The heart stores the *shen* or spirit, and is therefore considered to be the seat of consciousness and mental functions. If the heart is working normally, and qi and blood are abundant, the mind is lucid, alert, and responsive to the environment (Wiseman & Feng 1998).

Mental illnesses and emotional disorders in general affect the heart, but rather than originating in the heart itself, damage by the emotions begins in some other viscus or bowel eventually affecting the heart (Schnyer & Flaws 1998). All emotions affect the heart besides affecting their corresponding viscus or bowel (Maciocia 1994). Many of the symptoms characteristic of mental and emotional imbalance, such as sleep disturbances, incoherent speech, confusion and disorientation, anxiety and palpitations, correspond to an inability of the heart to perform the function of housing the *shen*. The heart's ability to house the spirit can be affected by disease mechanisms that precipitate either vacuity or repletion patterns. When we refer throughout this manual to the concept of *shen disturbance*, we are referring to the different patterns that affect the heart's function of housing the *shen* or spirit.

Spleen

> 'The Spleen and Stomach are responsible for the storehouses and granaries. The five Wei (tastes) stem from them.' (Su Wen, Ch. 8; cited in Larre & Rochat de la Vallée 1985, p. 64)

The spleen assimilates nutrients from food in the stomach to make qi, blood, and fluids; it governs the movement and transformation of food and water and the distribution of its essence (nutrients), playing a very important role in the creation of qi and blood. In Chinese Medicine it is said that the spleen is the source of qi and blood formation (Wiseman & Feng 1998), the source of engenderment and transformation (Schnyer & Flaws 1998). On the one hand, if the spleen becomes diseased it may not be able to create and transform sufficient qi and blood to nurture the heart and to provide mental clarity and awareness. On the other hand, if it fails in its function of moving and transforming body fluids, dampness may accumulate and lead to phlegm. Phlegm in Chinese Medicine denotes a viscous (yin) fluid that, when accumulated, may cause disease anywhere in the body; it may create a disturbance of the heart spirit and affect mental functions characterized by confused thinking, dullness of thought, brooding, and rumination.

Lung

> 'The Lung holds the office of Minister and Chancellor. The regulation of the life-giving network stems from it.' (Su Wen, Ch. 8; cited in Larre & Rochat de la Vallée 1985, p. 30)

The lung is responsible for breathing and the production of qi; it moves and circulates the qi out to the edges of the body and from the top downwards. It assists the metabolism of body fluids by carrying water downwards to the bladder and preventing the accumulation of water in the body. In addition, the lung helps to protect the body from invasion by external pathogens. Like the heart, the lung is often affected by disease processes initiated in other viscera and bowels. For example, when liver qi stagnation affects the lung, it may create a sense of constriction in the chest, breathlessness, and a tendency to weep.

Kidney

> 'The Kidneys are responsible for the creation of power. Skill and ability stem from them.' (Su Wen, Ch. 8; cited in Larre & Rochat de la Vallée 1985, p. 76)

As we saw previously, the kidney as a single functional unit provides the basis for our congenital constitution; it stores the essence and holds the foundation for the yin and yang of all other viscera and bowels. The essential qi of the kidney is responsible not only for our reproductive capacity but also for the growth, development, and aging of the body (Wiseman & Feng 1998). In addition, any enduring disease damages the kidney, including mental and emotional problems. The harmonious relationship between the kidney and the heart is fundamental for the physical and mental wellbeing of the organism; these two viscera are interdependent and counterbalance each other. The kidney is the seat of the essence (*jing*), while the heart is the abode of the spirit (*shen*). Jing and shen, essence and spirit, soma and psyche, are aspects of a continuous process. *Shen* refers to the organizing force of the self, whereas *jing* refers to the material substance; together they refer to the totality of the human being (Beinfield & Korngold 1991).

Gall Bladder

'The Gall Bladder is responsible for what is just and exact. Determination and decision stem from it.' (Su Wen, Ch. 8; cited in Larre & Rochat de la Vallée 1985, p. 43)

The main functions of the gall bladder are to secrete bile, which is formed from an excess of liver qi, and to govern decision. This last function implies that the capacity to maintain a balanced judgement in the face of adversity is attributed to this bowel; strong gall bladder qi ensures less vulnerability to external stimuli (Wiseman & Feng 1998), greater courage, and less timidity.

The gall bladder, however, plays a very important and somewhat peculiar role in the clinical treatment of mental–emotional disorders. This role is based on the relationship that the gall bladder has to the heart on the one hand, and to the liver on the other. The 11 organs are said to depend on the gall bladder and, therefore, if the qi of the gall bladder is strong, endogenous or exogenous pathogens cannot enter. These two statements link the gall bladder to the heart and its spirit, and elevate it to a place of greater importance (Schnyer & Flaws 1998). The relationship between the heart and the gall bladder is further emphasized by a Chinese Medicine theory known as the 'midday–midnight law'. This theory states that the circulation of qi along the channels is said to take its course over a period of 24 hours; according to this theory there is a special clinical relationship between viscera and bowels, which receive their maximal flow at opposite times of the day (Mann 1973). The heart has its maximal activity at 12 noon, while the gall bladder has its maximum activity at 12 midnight.[5] If the gall bladder is stimulated through acupuncture, the heart will be stimulated as well. It is interesting to note in this regard that several acupuncture points located on the gall bladder channel have a very profound effect on the treatment of mental–emotional conditions. Furthermore, the gall bladder is considered 'the official residence of clear fluids' (Flaws 1994) and it influences the transformation of body fluids. Therefore, points along the gall bladder channel are very effective in the treatment of patterns that involve accumulation of dampness and phlegm obstructing mental clarity, which are frequently found in depression. It is also worth mentioning that the guiding herbal prescription traditionally used to treat these type of patterns (phlegm dampness, obstruction, and stagnation, phlegm confounding the orifices of the heart, heart vacuity–gall

[5]This theory goes on to say that, when a viscus or bowel is stimulated, the viscus or bowel that it is connected to though the 'midday–midnight law' is actually stimulated in the opposite sense, i.e. if the gall bladder is supplemented, the heart is actually drained (Mann 1973).

bladder timidity, and phlegm fire harassing the heart) is known as 'warm the gall bladder decoction' (*wen dan tang*).

Also, the gall bladder stands as the yang counterpart of the liver. When qi (which is yang) accumulates, it becomes hot and tends to move in a yang direction: upwards. Therefore, stagnant liver qi commonly moves into its paired yang channel, the gall bladder; symptoms of liver depression qi stagnation commonly appear along the course of the gall bladder channel as fullness, distension and lack of free flow (Schnyer & Flaws 1998).

Stomach

The stomach is the first to receive foods and liquids into the body; it is in the stomach that foods and liquids are first collected and are broken down to allow their nutrients to be absorbed. In complementary opposition to the spleen, which extracts the nutrients from food and sends them up to the lungs to be distributed, the stomach sends the food down to the intestines to be further absorbed and eliminated. In Chinese Medicine it is said that the *spleen upbears the clear* and the *stomach downbears the turbid* to explain this complementary relationship. Together with the spleen, the stomach has a pivotal role in the creation of qi and blood; many of the disease mechanisms responsible for depression due to insufficiency of qi and blood are a result of disturbance in the functions of both the stomach and the spleen. In repletion patterns it is very common to find stagnant liver qi attacking the stomach and upsetting its downbearing function, and for liver heat to collect in the stomach. Liver depression qi stagnation can render both the stomach and the spleen incapable of performing their respective functions. On the one hand the stomach becomes 'dry and hot' and cannot downbear the turbid, while the spleen becomes 'damp and weak' and cannot upbear the clear. In addition, because the heart is said to be located above the stomach in Chinese Medicine and, because heat tends to rise, stomach heat counterflows upwards and agitates the heart (Schnyer & Flaws 1998).

Functions of the Viscera and Bowels and their Role in Depression

Depression, as well as any other mood disorder, can be a manifestation of an imbalance in certain functions of the viscera and bowels. Emotions are considered to be manifestations of qi that, if not expressed or transformed, become stagnant; they become a cause of disease only when they are experienced excessively or for a prolonged period of time, or both (Maciocia 1994). When the qi does not circulate properly, it becomes noxious and generates an imbalance.

Chinese Medicine does not separate physiological and psychological events; the *shen* or spirit is made by both qi and blood, which in turn are generated by the viscera and bowels. At the same time, the functions of the viscera and bowels, our qi, and our spirit are affected by external circumstances. In Schnyer & Flaws (1998), Bob Flaws explains it in this way: 'the mind arises as a function of the viscera and bowels, but the functioning of the viscera and bowels is affected by the experiences of the mind and the emotions' (p. 15). He goes on to say: 'every thought or felt emotion is nothing other than the experience of the movement of qi ... [C]hanging the way the qi moves, one changes one's mental–emotional experience, while changing one's mind and emotions changes the way the qi moves' (p. 15).

The lung, spleen, and kidney (particularly the yang aspect of the kidney) are the viscera more directly involved in the production and transformation of our qi; the quality and quantity of qi depends on their functions. Therefore these viscera are most likely involved in patterns of depression due to vacuity of qi/yang or accumulation of dampness and phlegm. Owing to the role the liver plays in maintaining the free movement of qi (and blood), it will likely be involved in patterns resulting from qi stagnation, although the stagnation may also directly affect the heart and lungs. The surplus of qi generated by liver depression qi stagnation can, over time, when severe or when combined with predisposing factors, create a predominance of yang (heat or fire). Yang repletion may accumulate in the liver, the heart or the stomach, and it may also consume yin, primarily of the liver, the kidney, and the heart. Liver depression qi stagnation may also progress into blood stasis, or it may generate accumulation of dampness or phlegm. Shen disturbance can be a result of either vacuity or repletion disease mechanisms that stem from dysfunction in other viscera and bowels; shen disturbance implies an imbalance in the heart's function of housing the *shen* or spirit (see Table 3.1).

The most important viscera associated with the mechanism of depression are the liver, heart, and spleen; however, the kidney and lung also play important roles. The gall bladder and the stomach are the only two bowels that have special significance in depression. In brief, we will look at the role of each of these viscera and bowels in the precipitation of depressive episodes.

ASSESSMENT AND TREATMENT FRAMEWORK

Acupuncture is said to adjust the density and flow of qi in the channels and network vessels, which in turn affects the circulation of other vital substances (blood and body fluids) and the function of the viscera and bowels. Chinese medical theory, as it relates to acupuncture, encompasses five areas that provide the framework for assessment and treatment (Seem 1987). These areas are:

1. Eight guiding criteria
2. Qi, blood, and body fluids
3. The viscera and bowels
4. The channels and network vessels
5. The five phases.

Based on the training and style of the practitioner, one of these areas may be used primarily or several may be used in combination. We have explained in some detail some of the basic theoretical concepts that serve as the foundation for the aforementioned assessment areas. We now describe how the information gathered by examination is then organized using each one of these assessment areas as 'filters', through which we interpret the information.

The Eight Principles

The eight principles or eight guiding criteria are four sets of bipolar categories that help to differentiate and interpret the information gathered during examination (Beinfield & Korngold 1991). They serve as a conceptual matrix that enables the practitioner to organize the relationship between particular clinical signs and yin and yang (Kaptchuk 1983). Disease patterns can be identified by means of these eight fundamental principles: *interior–exterior, cold–heat, vacuity–repletion* and *yin–yang*. They determine the relative location, nature, and quality of the imbalance and constitute the basis of differential diagnosis from which the patterns of disharmony evolve. Interior and exterior describe depth of the disease; cold and heat describe the nature of the disease; vacuity and repletion describe the relative strength or weakness of one's own right qi in relationship to pathogenic qi; yin and yang are the general categories that embrace the other six principles (Wiseman & Feng 1998). Interior, cold, and vacuity are yin features, whereas exterior, heat, and repletion are yang features. Each principle is associated with specific signs; by matching the patient's signs the depth and nature of the diseases can be determined, as well as the relative strength of the forces that resist the disease and those that cause it (Wiseman & Feng 1998).

Seem (1987) developed a phenomenological model that explains the mechanism for the development of vacuity and repletion patterns of either yin or yang, depending on one's constitutional tendencies of 'becoming hot' (yang) or 'becoming cold' (yin) (Fig. 3.1). According to Seem's model, we can interpret disease patterns as 'somatic energetic reaction patterns' that develop along one of two continua: *yin deficiency–yang excess* (hyperactivity and increased metabolic response) or *yang deficiency–yin excess* (hypoactivity, decreased metabolic response). In this view, when confronted with an emotional stressor or a perceived threat, the organism would tend to react in one of two ways: by activating sympathetic response in preparation for 'fight or flight' (yang) or by withdrawing from external activity and parasympathetically attending to internal demands and allowing the organism to 'rest and digest' (yin). If sympathetic activation is prolonged, the organism exists in a chronic state of readiness, with the corresponding physiological reactions. Yang overtakes yin. If, on the other hand, the response is parasympathetic, the body will withdraw from action into a dependent stage, retreating from danger and looking for help. Yin overtakes yang (Seem 1987).[6]

We can use this interpretation of eight principles pattern differentiation to establish a parallel between these two reaction tendencies and the various symptoms of major depression. As shown in Table 3.1, each of the DSM-IV symptoms of major depression has corresponding symptoms of vacuity and repletion (deficiency/excess) of either yin or yang.

Qi, Blood, and Body Fluids

The mechanisms for the generation, transformation, and movement of qi, blood, and body fluids, which we explained above, are used as the conceptual matrix to understand the interactions and manifestations of yin and yang in the human body. Yin and yang are water and fire in the world, whereas qi and blood are fire and water in the body (Schnyer & Flaws 1998). As seen earlier, body fluids are also either yin or yang, depending on their function and nature. Essence and spirit also form a complementary yin and yang pair.

---

[6]As we can see in Figure 3.1, if the yin of the kidney becomes situated on the left side of the five phases diagram, and the yang of the kidney on the right, when the yin of the kidney is vacuous or deficient 'becoming hot' tendencies develop along the phases (and associated viscera) that are on the left; and 'becoming cold' tendencies due to yang vacuity develop along the phases (and viscera) on the right.

FIGURE 3.1 *A phenomenological model for understanding the development of patterns.*

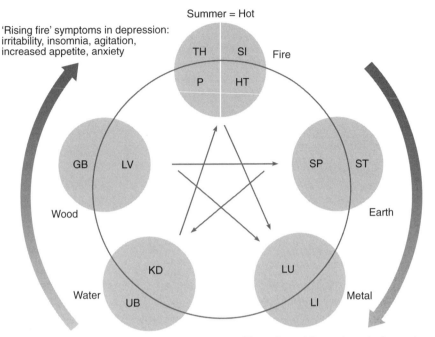

This figure shows basic tendencies towards yin or yang functioning. When the yin of the kidney is situated on the left side of the five phases diagram, and the yang of the kidney is situated on the right side, kidney yin vacuity tendencies ('becoming hot') develop in the viscera and bowels, which are situated on the left side of the diagram (wood and fire). These tendencies manifest as rising heat disorders of the liver, gall bladder and heart. Similarly, when the yang of the kidney is vacuous, 'becoming cold' tendencies develop in the viscera and bowels on the right side of the chart (earth and metal), with cold disorders in the stomach and spleen, and dampness–phlegm accumulation in the spleen and lungs. GB, gall bladder; HT, heart; KD, kidney; LI, large intestine; LU, lung; LV, liver; P, pericardium; SI, small intestine; SP, spleen; ST, stomach; TH, triple heater; UB, urinary bladder. Adapted with kind permission from Seem (1987).

Clinically, when using qi, blood, and body fluids as a diagnostic filter, one determines the relative insufficiency or accumulation of qi and blood, the quality of generation, movement, and transformation of body fluids, and the condition and presence of the essence and spirit. In addition, the clinician evaluates the functional interactions between the viscera and bowels responsible with the production and movement of these 'substances'. The use of qi, blood, and body fluids as a theoretical framework, in conjunction with the eight principles and the viscera and bowels, together constitute the foundation for TCM as a style of treatment.

TABLE 3.2		*The 71 channels*			
No. of channels	Name	Type of qi carried	Characteristics	Functions	Strategies that best address each level
12	Tendinomuscular	Protective (wei)	1. Site of exogenous invasion 2. Bodymind's character armor	1. *Acute reaction patterns:* as reaction to stressors 2. *Chronic reaction patterns:* as part of a series of reactions of the bodymind. Always the same points and meridians	1. Musculoskeletal 2. Bi-syndromes 3. Trigger points 4. Six great units 5. Eight extra meridians
12	Regular	Nourishing (ying)	1. Connection between structure and function (surface of the body with viscera and bowels) 2. Functional energetics: a. metaphors of function/dysfunction b. constitutional factors c. coping factors d. behavioral reaction patterns	1. Behavior at somatic energetic level: stress responses as an insult to function 2. Organ inferiorities. (predisposition to disease)	1. Functions and dysfunctions of channels and viscera and bowels 2. Bodymind: a. Eight principles b. Five phases
8	Extraordinary	Essence (jing)	1. Core energetics: essential procreative energies of jing and *shen*, essence and spirit, soma and psyche 2. Rooted in the energetic center: hara/ming-men 3. Transformation of no-form into pre- and postnatal energies	Divide the body in eight areas: a) Left and right (du/re mo) b) Upper and lower (daimo) c) Front and back of yang (yang wei/ yang chiao mo) d) Front and back of yin (yin wei/yin chiao mo)	1. Expressed in body balance and symmetry 2. Intimately related to structure 3. Reflected in the hara
12	Connecting	Nourishing (ying)	1. Provide a crossover network between coupled channels, one yin and one yang 2. Carry qi from one channel to the next, in a process in which the qi is transformed from yin into yang and vice versa	They join each pair of channels, yin and yang	Luo points

No. of channels	Name	Type of qi carried	Characteristics	Functions	Strategies that best address each level
14	Linking (luo)	Nourishing (ying)	12 for one of each regular, and one each for du mai and ren mai	1. Extend the influence of the main channels to other parts of the body 2. Constitute a reservoir of qi between the regular channel and its respective viscus or bowel 3. Act as a buffer that absorbs excess qi from the regular channels	Luo points
1	Great linking	Nourishing (ying)		Connects all the linking (luo) channels	Sp 21
12	Divergent	Nourishing (ying)	Leave the main channels at various points, but do not rejoin them; instead they join their coupled yang channel	They are considered of equal importance to the regular channels	Divergent channel points

Source: Seem (1990).

Channels and Network Vessels

The network of channels in the human body is composed by four major systems: (1) the 12 regular channels, (2) the eight extraordinary vessels, (3) the secondary vessels, which include the tendinomuscular, connecting, and linking channels, and (4) the divergent channels. There are, in total, 71 channels (see Table 3.2) (Seem 1990).

There are various approaches to using the channels and network vessels as a filter. For example, one may focus on knowing which level – defensive, nourishing, ancestral – is affected, in order to treat the corresponding network (Seem 1990). Alternatively, one may emphasize the treatment of the areas irrigated by the channels, as zones that are said to be structured and organized by the particular influence of each channel (Seem 1993). One may also use the concept of the six great units as constitutional diathesis (predisposition to disease) based on Yves Requena's (1986) approach. The framework used throughout this manual incorporates these last two concepts: (1) the influence of the channels on different areas of the body when making our final point selection and (2) the six great units as constitutional diathesis, for understanding predisposition to the different pattern combinations.

The Channel System

The 12 Regular Channels

The 12 regular channels form the basic structure of the channel system and provide a network of qi and blood by which the whole body is nourished (Wiseman & Feng 1998). There are six yin and six yang channels, three of each on each hand and three of each on each foot. Each channel homes to viscera and bowels that stand in an interior–exterior (yin–yang) relationship. In addition to being paired by their internal–external relationship (yin–yang), the regular channels are also paired by the same polarity (yin or yang), with one arm channel and one leg channel to form the six great units; this results in a complex set of interactions that allow the acupuncturist to make subtle interventions to restore balance. Figure 3.2 lists the names of the 12 regular channels, their abbreviations, and their relationships.

The Eight Extraordinary Vessels

The eight extraordinary vessels are thought to develop prenatally before the development of the main channels; their function is to supplement insufficiencies of the other channels. The extraordinary channels do not home to any organs and do not have an interior–exterior relationship; they connect channels of the same polarity, whether yin or yang (Wiseman & Feng 1998). The extraordinary channels are du mai, ren mai, chong mai, dai mai, yang wei mai, yin wei mai, yang chao mai, and yin chao mai.

The Secondary Vessels

The secondary vessels include the tendinomuscular channels, the connecting and the linking channels. The tendinomuscular channels run parallel to the regular channels on the surface of the body. The linking channels (*luo*) include 12 channels for each regular channel, plus one for du mai and one for ren mai. They extend the influence of the main channels to other parts of the body (Low 1983).

FIGURE 3.2   *The 12 regular channels: internal–external relationship and the six units*

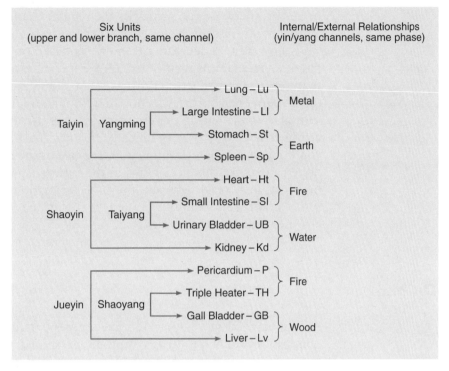

Two relationships between the channels are shown: in the right-hand column, the internal–external or yin–yang relationship is highlighted: one viscus and one bowel of the same phase are paired. On the left-hand side, the relationship that corresponds to the six units, between the upper and lower branches of each channel, is emphasized. This relationship underlines the correspondence between the viscus or bowel of one phase, with the viscus or bowel of a different phase. Adapted with kind permission from Seem (1987).

The Divergent Channels

The divergent channels leave the main channels at various points, but do not rejoin them; instead they join their coupled yang channel (Low 1983). They are considered of equal importance to the regular channels.

The channels are said to develop from conception through adulthood; each channel level is said to carry a different kind of qi: defensive (*wei*), nourishing (*ying*), and ancestral (*jing*) (Seem 1990). The first to develop are three of the extraordinary vessels (du mai, ren mai, and chong mai; see below); then comes dai mai, followed by the remaining four extraordinary vessels. The second set of channels to develop are the tendinomuscular, followed by the regular, and finally the connecting, linking, and divergent pathways. For a summary of the different channel levels and their functions, see Figure 3.2.

Channels and Network Vessels in the Treatment of Depression

In our protocol, we use primarily the regular channels because we are aiming at addressing dysfunction of the viscera and bowels. It is possible, however, to develop a framework based on addressing the different channel levels mentioned above; it can be argued, for example, that depression is a stress response that should be treated initially at the level of the character armor (tendinomuscular level), or that one should aim at treating the core through the use of the extraordinary channels (Seem 1990). Clinically, it may be extremely useful to combine, in a progressive fashion, the use of the different levels. We hope to explore this possibility in the future. The present approach, however, involves solely outlining the rationale for the inclusion of some point combinations aimed at balancing two extraordinary channels, du mai and chong mai.

Du Mai

As summarized in Chapter 1, some studies conducted in China used points along du mai to treat symptoms associated with depression. Du mai, or the governing channel, plays a very important role in depression. Du mai is one of the eight extraordinary channels and does not have a corresponding viscera or bowel. It emerges from the kidney; it is the storehouse of the yang, the sea of the yang channels, and has a regulating effect on the yang qi of the whole body. It begins its pathway at the perineum and ascends along the spine, up over the head and into the mouth. It is said in Chinese Medicine that the governing vessel homes to the brain and nets the kidney. Since the kidney engenders the marrow and the brain is known as the 'sea of marrow', the governing vessel reflects the physiology and pathology of the brain and the spinal fluid, as well as their relationship to the reproductive organs (Wiseman & Feng 1998). The points along its pathway have been used traditionally, among other things, to affect mental functions. An excess of qi along the channel would mean an exuberance of yang: too much energy traveling 'upward' towards the head or stuck in the upper part of the body creating irritability, restlessness, and insomnia. An insufficiency in the flow of qi along its pathway will result in the inability of total yang of the organism to circulate, raise, and nourish the brain and spinal cord, manifesting as apathy, flat affect, and inability to express enthusiasm or emotion. The section on point indications provides greater detail on how we have used du mai in our protocol.

Chong Mai

Chong mai is where all the qi and blood of the 12 regular channels converge and it is considered to have a regulating effect on all of them (Wiseman & Feng 1998). The transportation and movement of the qi and blood of the whole body is focused on the chong, and therefore it is called the 'sea of blood' (Flaws 1997). The chong mai arises from the kidney and connects the liver with the pericardium (*jueyin*), bringing together the functions of menstruation (liver) and reproduction (kidney) with the heart's function of housing the spirit. Chong mai is traditionally indicated in the treatment of menstrual and gynecological disorders, and it is broadly used to treat morning sickness during pregnancy.

In its pathway, the chong mai raises up through the regions irrigated by the liver and kidney (yin), connecting the peritoneum, the pleura, and the pericardium, and serving as the foundation upon which all the functions of the viscera and bowels develop (Seem 1990). The chong mai comprises the entire visceral cavity, and integrates the areas primarily affected by stagnation of liver qi.

The liver rules the area of the diaphragm and the region of the ribs. When confronted with a stressor, one commonly tightens up the diaphragm as well as the musculature of the chest and the upper back, the throat, the jaw, and the head. If this constriction of the diaphragm develops into a chronic stress response, the upper and lower regions of the body become 'split', as if one was cut off, so to speak, at the diaphragm, leaving the lower parts of the body vacuous and weak (kidney yang vacuity) and creating hyperactivity and agitation in the upper parts of the body (shen disturbance). In people experiencing depression, it is very common to find a constriction in the diaphragm, and neck and shoulder tension (liver qi stagnation), in combination with symptoms of decreased metabolic response on the one hand (kidney yang vacuity) and anxiety and agitation (yin vacuity–hyperactivity of yang) on the other. Chong mai allows us to integrate the complex relationship of patterns found in depression that involve the liver, the heart, the spleen, and the kidney simultaneously.

The Five Phases

The relationship between yin and yang is further differentiated into identifiable stages that describe the process of change between situations and across time. These stages – *wood*, *fire*, *earth*, *metal*, and *water* – are known as the *five phases* and reflect the transformation of yin into yang, and vice versa. Like yin and yang, the five phases are

TABLE 3.3	Correspondence between the five phases, viscera and bowels, psychological and physiological functions, and their relationship to DSM-IV depression				
	Wood	**Fire**	**Earth**	**Metal**	**Water**
Organ network	Liver (gall bladder)	Heart (small intestine)	Spleen (stomach)	Lung (large intestine)	Kidney (bladder)
Emotions and their imbalances	Anger Qi tends to raise, lash out or, if unexpressed, become stagnant	Joy or fright Qi tends to get dissipated and scattered	Worry or pensiveness Excessive thinking and rumination cause the qi to bind	Sorrow Inability to overcome grief weakens our qi and cuts us away from life	Fear Qi tends to descend or becomes petrified and frozen
Physiological functions	Regulate movement of qi, store and distribute the blood	Propel the blood; house the *shen* or spirit. Maintain awareness	Extract nutrients from food, transform them into qi and blood, and distribute them	Establish basic rhythm of organism and incorporate the qi through respiration	Generate and store essence; govern reproduction; balance fluids
Physiological dysfunctions	Stagnation of qi and stasis of blood, pain, distension, menstrual or digestive irregularities	Circulatory problems, anxiety, agitation or nervous exhaustion	Lethargy, indigestion, appetite disturbances, water retention	Respiratory disorders, shallow breathing, lack of energy or motivation	Loss of libido, reproductive disorders, chronic back pain
Psychological functions	Evenness of emotion, consistent behavior	Expression and integration of our being	Assimilation of experiences and incorporation of them into who we are	Set limits, protect boundaries, distinguish past from present	Conserve resources in times of growth, crises, transition
Psychological features	Emotive Organizes around change, action, challenge, solutions, independence	Sensitive Organizes around realization, fulfillment, intimacy, desire, pleasure	Reflective Organizes around unification, harmony, community, pleasing others	Deductive Organizes around refinement, order, principles of reason, standards	Instinctive Organizes around knowledge, truth, ideas, introspection
Mental aspect	Hun: Provides us with proper judgement, vision, insight, intuition: gives us sense of direction; allows us to plan; influences sleep and dreaming	Shen: Maintains our awareness and expresses the total expression and integration of our being	Yi: Provides concentration and memorization. When imbalanced we tend to think constantly, to brood and ruminate	Po: Serves as organizational principle of the body, giving us the capacity of movement, agility and coordination	Zhi: Responsible for drive, determination and long-term memory
Possible precipitating features for depression	Inability to modulate intensity and stay flexible	Difficulty tempering fervor and conserving own resources	Dependent on being needed by others, insists on predictability, security and loyalty	Over-rigidity, self-control, indifference, self-righteousness, and disillusionment	Emotionally inaccessible, undemonstrative, tactless, unforgiving, suspicious
DSM-IV associated features	Depression with irritability, periodic outburst of anger, frustration; erratic physical complaints; digestive disturbance	Depression with diminished interest and pleasure; insomnia, anxiety, speech disturbances, diminished ability to think or concentrate, feelings of worthlessness	Depression with lethargy, excessive, or inappropriate guilt, rumination, apathy, phobias	Depression with lethargy and weakness, psychomotor retardation, fatigue	Depression with lethargy, apathy, decreased libido, isolation

Source: Beinfeld & Korngold (1991).

categories of quality and relationship (Wiseman & Feng 1998). Change is a process that takes place gradually as qi moves around the cycle represented by the five phases. According to the five phases theory, phenomena in the universe are the result of the movement and mutation of these five entities. Wood, fire, earth, metal, and water represent certain qualities and relate to one another in specific ways; any other group of five phenomena that have qualities and relate to each other in similar ways are said to correspond to the five phases (Wiseman & Feng 1998; see also Table 3.3).

Yin, which expresses the potential of the bodymind (i.e. totality of soma and psyche), is characterized by *water*, and corresponds to the apparent quiescent stasis of the winter – a time when, beneath the surface, germination is preparing to bring forth the renewal of spring. It represents the capacity to store, generate, charge, and restore after release (Beinfield & Korngold 1991). 'Water is the moistening and descending to low places' (p. 206); it corresponds to the blackness of the night, and with saltiness, the taste of sea water (Wiseman & Feng 1998).

Fire characterizes yang, the dynamic principle, the sense of splendor and fulfillment experienced when light, warmth, and interaction are at their peak. Fire symbolizes the end point of expansion and consummation, of completion and fulfillment (Beinfield & Korngold 1991). 'Fire is the flaming upward, and has the quality and upward movement' (p. 205); it is associated with summer, with the color red, and the bitter taste (Wiseman & Feng 1998).

The transition of yin (the seed and the root) into yang (the flower and fruit) is represented by *wood*, an ascending movement of sudden growth and rapid expansion, of unexpected but unpredictable change (Beinfield & Korngold 1991). 'Wood is the bending and the straightening' (p. 205), it grows upward and stretches outward; it corresponds to the spring, the time of growth and the beginning of the cycle of the seasons, it is associated with the green of new leaves in the sour taste of unripe fruit (Wiseman & Feng 1998). When the life force reaches its greatest expression, it begins to slow down, collapsing inward.

Metal represents the capacity for separation and refinement that is expressed in the autumn, when the energy contracts in order to consolidate, when the leaves fall and fertilize the soil for the next spring (Beinfield & Korngold 1991). 'Metal is the working of change' (p. 206), having the qualities of purification, elimination, and reform; it is associated with the white color of frost, and with the purifying action of acrid smelling things (Wiseman & Feng 1998).

These processes happen as we find ourselves on the *earth*, the point of reference that locates us in time and space. Earth represents our capacity for changing direction without losing balance, and is the axis around which other aspects orient themselves (Beinfield & Korngold

1991). 'Earth is the sowing and reaping' (p. 206), representing the planting and harvesting of crops and the bringing forth of phenomena. Earth is associated with yellow (the Chinese word includes brown), and with the sweetness of ripened fruit (Wiseman & Feng 1998).

Clinically, the five phases constitute a system for understanding the movement of qi through the five viscera; each of the five viscera corresponds to each of the five phases. Wiseman & Feng (1998) illustrate the relationship between the functions of the five viscera and the qualities of the five phases as follows:

> 'The liver controls the movement of qi around the body; it spreads qi just as the trees spread their branches; and as trees and other plants sprout upwards in the spring, so the liver yang tends to stir upwards. The heart has the function of propelling qi and blood to warm and nourish the whole body; it is like a fire that drives the body, just like the heat of summer makes nature flourish. The spleen is the source of qi and blood, that nourish and drive the body, just like the earth brings forth the crops at the end of the summer. The lung helps transform the fluids into blood, it controls the downward movement of the fluids to the kidney and bladder, and in this way is responsible for the purifying removal of waste fluids; it has the purifying qualities of the autumn frost. The kidney stores essence, just as nature preserves itself in winter dormancy.' (Wiseman & Feng 1998, p. 206)

The five phases explain the etiology and nature of qi imbalances, providing in this way the framework for an energetic physiology to further comprehend the disturbances of the bodymind (Seem 1987). In addition to having similar qualities to one another, the phenomena associated with the five phases relate to other phenomena associated with the same phase in a similar fashion; for example, water engenders wood, and winter gives way to spring, and so the kidney (water) nourishes the liver (wood). Each phase corresponds to a set of channels and to a viscus and a bowel paired by their yin–yang relationship. (Each paired system is commonly identified by the name of the yin function: liver–wood, heart–fire, spleen–earth, metal–lung, water–kidney.)

According to Beinfield & Korngold (1991), every viscus and bowel has a responsibility or job to do, a strategy on how to do the job, and a character or way to do it, which reflects the nature of the energy represented by its pertaining phase. Every phase characteristically influences physiological and psychological functions that in turn correspond to the particular viscus (and bowel) associated with it. There is a corresponding tissue, sense, body fluid, sound, and smell associated with each phase, as shown in Box 3.3. In addition there is an emotion and a mental aspect associated with each of the five phases. A more comprehensive description of the correspondence between

BOX 3.3	Correspondences of the five phases				
	Wood	**Fire**	**Earth**	**Metal**	**Water**
	Liver	Heart	Spleen	Lung	Kidney
	Tendons and ligaments	Blood vessels	Muscles and flesh	Skin and body hair	Bones and head hair
	Sight	Speech	Taste	Smell	Hearing
	Tears	Blood	Saliva	Sweat	Urine
	Shout	Laugh	Sing	Weep	Groan
	Rancid	Scorched	Fragrant	Rotten	Putrid

the five phases, the five viscera, the emotions, and the mental aspects associated with each one of them is given in 'The seven affects and the five emotions' and 'The five spirits' sections below.

In the context of the five phases, depression can be considered an imbalance in the movement of qi along the cycle of transformation of the energy. The five phases interact with one another according to patterns of generation and restraint which explain their capacity and provide the motivating impulse for their potential (Beinfield & Korngold 1991). Illness is considered a process, not a static entity. When using the five phases as the basis for diagnosis and treatment, the system of correspondences is used to identify constitutional tendencies and to determine the configuration presented by the interaction of signs and symptoms, in order to attend to the root of the patient's imbalance. Emotional disturbances are well explained using the theory of the five phases as a framework, which makes it an especially useful tool to understand distinct constitutional predispositions to depression, to reframe the symptoms experienced by the person, and to develop a model for patient education. In the section on Assessment in Chapter 5 we will describe how the five phases have been used in the protocol presented in this manual. The correspondence between the five phases, the five viscera, and the etiology and symptom presentation of major depression are also detailed in Table 3.3.

EMOTIONS AND QI: THE BODYMIND CONTINUUM

The Seven Affects and the Five Emotions

As seen above, each of the five phases and its corresponding viscus has an associated emotion. These five emotions – *anger, joy, worry, sadness,* and *fear* – are considered to be manifestations of qi, basic forms of emotional activity; they become a cause of disease only when experienced excessively, for a prolonged period of time, or both (Maciocia 1994). Two emotions, anxiety or oppression, and fright, are added to these five to complement the gamete of human emotions; together they constitute the seven affects. Oppression reinforces other emotions such as sadness, obsessive thinking, or fear; it represents contraction, lack of circulation, immobilization (Larre & Rochat de la Vallée 1996); sometimes translated as anxiety (Wiseman & Feng 1998), this emotion is attributed to the lung or spleen, depending on the context (Larre & Rochat de la Vallée 1996). Commonly, fright refers to being startled with fright, and can mean any movement of the body, such as shaking or convulsions; it corresponds to the liver. Table 3.3 provides a summary of the correspondence between the viscera, the five phases, and the emotions.

When disease originates from emotional causes it is known in Chinese Medicine as *internal damage*, *affect damage*, or *damage by the emotions*.[7]

When the emotions are experienced persistently or intensely, they can alter the balance between yin and yang, blood and qi, and adversely affect the functions of the viscera and bowels. For example, whereas the liver, heart, and spleen seem to be involved most directly with the core symptoms of major depression, the interactions of these with other viscera and bowels can play a role in the appearance of other physical and psychological symptoms that may be seen during depression. These are symptoms for which depressed individuals may visit a physician, only to find no medical basis for their complaints. Because all symptoms, both physiological and psychological, are relevant in Chinese Medicine, these additional symptoms are equally important in determining the pattern of disharmony underlying depression. These symptoms help to establish the diagnosis and selection of treatment principles and points.

For example, anger causes the qi to rise and can create distension and fullness in the rib cage and breasts, headaches, dizziness, and red, sore eyes; because the liver stores the blood, ascendant liver qi may carry the blood with it and cause nose bleeding. Because the liver and the spleen are closely related through the control cycle of the five phases, excessive liver qi moves across, 'attacks' and affects the spleen, making it incapable of performing its functions of transportation and transformation. A very common scenario encountered in depressive episodes is *liver qi stagnation* (frustration, irritability) in conjunction

---

[7]In Chinese Medicine, disease is said to originate from one of three causes: internal, external, or neutral (neither internal nor external). The emotions are said to be the internal causes of disease and are not to be confused with evils that arise internally such as internal fire or internal wind, which may develop from affect damage, but which can also be the result of insufficiency or transformation of external evils (Wiseman & Feng 1998).

with a weak spleen, or *spleen vacuity* (weight changes, worry, abdominal distension); this weakness of spleen may, in turn, generate *dampness or phlegm accumulation* (*yin repletion*). Anger can also affect the stomach (nausea/vomiting), large intestine (irritable bowel), lungs (coughing and wheezing), and heart (agitation, insomnia).

Joy causes the qi to slacken; excessive joy leads to a dissipation of *shen*, or spirit, and a weakening of the heart qi, manifesting as heart palpitations, insomnia, and some mental diseases (Wiseman & Feng 1998) such as mania. Worry and overthinking cause the qi to bind, affecting movement and transportation and causing shallow breathing, fullness in the chest (lungs) and stomach, poor appetite, abdominal distension, and loose stools. They can also cause neck and shoulder stiffness (gall bladder, liver) (Maciocia 1994).

Sadness (grief) corresponds to the lungs. It causes the qi to disperse and can deplete lung qi, which manifests with a weak voice, breathlessness, and weeping, or a feeling of constriction in the chest. According to Maciocia (1994), sadness may also affect the liver and create mental confusion, a lack of sense of direction, and an inability to plan; when held in for many years, it can affect the kidney and its regulation of fluid metabolism.

Incontinence or diarrhea may be caused by fear, which makes the qi descend and corresponds to the kidney. Fright, which in the summary above is associated with the heart, causes chaos and derangement of the qi, manifesting as disquietude of the spirit, and possibly more severe mental illness (Wiseman & Feng 1998).

Affect damage or damage by the emotions can originate from and/or give rise to vacuity or repletion patterns. Shen disturbance vacuity patterns manifest primarily as heart blood or heart yin vacuity, and to a lesser extent as heart qi vacuity; they generally stem from constitutional or circumstantial predisposition to qi and blood vacuity. Shen disturbance repletion patterns stem from either liver depression or spleen and kidney vacuity. When originating from liver depression, they manifest as qi stagnation affecting the heart, depressive heart agitating the spirit, or blood stasis blocking the heart's orifices; when stemming from spleen and kidney vacuity, they manifest as variety of patterns that derive from phlegm obstructing the orifices of the heart. A more detailed review of how patterns encountered in depression generally evolve is presented in Chapter 5.

The Five Spirits: Five Mental Aspects of the Bodymind

In addition to the spirit (*shen*), which is stored by the heart, each yin viscus houses a specific mental aspect of the human mind. The *shen* itself indicates consciousness and memory; it maintains our awareness and expresses the integration of our being. The liver stores the *hun*, usually translated as the ethereal soul. The *hun* is said to complement the functions of the *shen*, and it is related to intuition and inspiration, insight and courage. The hun gives us a sense of direction and the capacity for planning; it influences sleep and dreaming. In the spleen is stored the *yi* or reflection, which represents our verbally expressed thoughts, our capacity for applied thinking, studying, memorizing, focusing, concentrating, and generating ideas. The kidney stores the *zhi*, which corresponds to will, drive, and determination; it also provides us with the capacity to store information and is related to long-term memory. The *po* or corporeal soul is stored in the lung and is what gives the body its capacity for movement, physical sensation, and coordination. It can be linked to the physical expression of the *hun* or to the organizational principle of the body, and it is considered to be closely related to the essence, considered the foundation of human life.

Depending on the specific manifestations, severity, and precipitating factors in a depressive episode, one or more of these mental aspects will be affected. Table 3.3 includes a summary of these five mental aspects.

The Five Virtues and other Correspondences of the Five Phases

Any human quality, mental attribution, or emotional experience can be attributed to the five phases. For example, each of the five spirits has a primary responsibility for a particular virtue (Kaptchuk 2000). *Shen*, which resides in the heart and corresponds to fire, is responsible for ceremony and propriety (*li*). 'Propriety ensures that correct behavior fosters timely interactions and relationships' (Kaptchuk 2000, p. 64). *Hun*, which resides in the liver and corresponds to wood, is responsible for human kindness and benevolence (*ren*): 'it has an intimate relationship to a person's capacity to feel and endure pain' (Kaptchuk 2000, p. 61). In the spleen resides the *yi*, which corresponds to earth and is responsible for 'faithfulness, loyalty or sincerity (*xin*) and has the task of enabling and supporting new manifestations to come into being' (Kaptchuk 2000, p. 60). *Zhi*, which resides in the kidneys and corresponds to water, is responsible for the virtue of wisdom (*zhi*): 'a knowing that has to do with learning to have a relationship to what is unknown and what is unknowable ... a deep trust that the unknown eventually reveals an inevitable destiny' (Kaptchuk 2000, p. 62–63). In the lungs, which correspond to metal, resides the *po*. The *po* is responsible for the virtue of preciousness (*bao*). 'The *Po* is said to capture the perfection and completeness of a single moment or a short time span' (Kaptchuk 2000, p. 65).

In Chinese Medicine, virtue refers to impulse from which all things manifest through the movement of qi (Larre & Rochat de la Vallée 1995). In the *Ling Shu*, Chapter 8, it is said: 'Heaven in me is Virtue. Earth in me is Breaths. Virtue flows, Breaths spread out, and there is Life' (Larre & Rochat de la Vallée 1991a, p. 87). In the human being, 'virtue is the authenticity of the heart as it moves along', 'through virtue one both finds and possesses oneself', and 'virtue gives authenticity to the one that possesses virtue' (Larre & Rochat de la Vallée 1995). For a more complete interpretation of the five phases, their correspondences, and their clinical application, refer to the numerous books of Claude Larre & Elisabeth Rochat de la Vallée, such as *The Seven Emotions* and *Rooted in Spirit*, and to Harriette Beinfield & Efrem Korngold's *Between Heaven and Earth* and to Lonny S. Jarrett's *Nourishing Destiny*.

INTEGRATION OF THE FIVE FILTERS: A CLINICAL MODEL

Each of these five filters (the eight principles, qi, blood and body fluids, viscera and bowels, channels and network vessels and the five phases), when emphasized and used in certain combinations, constitute the basis for specific styles of acupuncture treatment. For example, when using them as 'filters' to interpret the information gathered through evaluation, the eight principles are generally combined with qi, blood and body fluids, and the viscera and bowels, to form a larger and more complete system. As discussed above, the theoretical framework that develops from the use of these three areas in combination constitutes the foundation for Traditional Chinese Medicine as a style of acupuncture treatment. Traditionally in TCM, the theory of the channels and network vessels is emphasized primarily to address dysfunctions of the viscera and bowels; the channels that most directly connect with the organs are the 12 regular channels. Therefore, within TCM, the use of these 12 channels with the addition of du mai and ren mai (known together as the 14 main channels) is considered to be sufficient for diagnosis and treatment (Schnyer & Flaws 1998). The use of the five phases theory in TCM focuses primarily on the correspondences between the five phases and the nature of the illness presented by the patient and, to some extent, on the selection and combination of acupuncture points. In the next chapter we describe the etiology of depression according to the eight guiding criteria and outline the specifics concerning the use of each filter in the treatment implementation.

The Etiology of Depression According to Traditional Chinese Medicine

OVERVIEW

Traditionally, psychiatric disease in Chinese Medicine is described by a single inclusive phrase of 'mania and withdrawal' (*dian kuang*). Mania denotes a state of excitement characterized by noisy, unruly, and possibly aggressive behavior (Wiseman & Feng 1998); it is due to hyperactivity of yang qi from any cause: heat that arises from qi stagnation, vacuity heat due to yin vacuity, fire transformation, etc. Withdrawal refers to emotional depression, indifference, no desire to eat or drink; it is a yin pattern in which yang is either not present because of qi or yang vacuity, or it is not flowing freely due to binding of depressed qi and phlegm (Wiseman & Feng 1998). Although classically the terms mania and withdrawal refer to severe forms of mental derangement, this classification is still valid in the treatment of unipolar depressive episodes even when not complicated by comorbidity or psychotic features.

DISEASE CAUSES AND MECHANISMS IN DEPRESSION

There are four concepts in Chinese Medicine that are extremely useful in understanding the progression of depression patterns, in differentiating conflicting signs and symptoms encountered in people experiencing depression, and in evaluating and treating complex pattern combinations. These four concepts are:

1. The concept of *qi stagnation*, its ramifications and complications

2. Zhu Dan-xi's theory of the *six depressions*
3. Liu Wan-su's theory of *similar transformation*
4. Li Dong-yuan's *yin fire* theory.

We were first introduced to these concepts through the teachings of Bob Flaws, especially as they applied to the treatment of gynecological and difficult-to-treat disorders. As we continued refining the treatment protocol for depression outlined in this manual, it became clear that these theories were fundamental in understanding the complex symptom pictures presented by our depressed patients. What follows is by no means a comprehensive description of these theories, but rather an overview of their relevance in the treatment of depression. For a more complete explanation of the theories presented below, please refer to the numerous writings of Bob Flaws cited in the bibliography. We will begin by explaining the six depressions and the theory of similar transformation, as these two theories help explain the progression of patterns that emerge from qi stagnation. We will describe then, in some detail, the mechanisms underlying qi stagnation patterns, and finally we will introduce the theory of yin fire.

The Six Depressions or Six Stagnations

The six depressions involve stagnation of either qi, blood, dampness, phlegm, food, or fire. Qi stagnation underlies all the others because qi is responsible for the movement and transformation of blood, dampness, phlegm, and food, and also because stagnant qi, being yang in nature, may eventually turn into fire or heat. Blood, dampness, phlegm, and food are all yin substances; if the qi becomes stagnant and depressed, it may result in any of these four not being moved or transformed properly, and they may accumulate (Flaws 1997). At the same time, the accumulation of any of these four yin substances may obstruct the free flow of yang qi, further complicating qi stagnation; the theory of similar transformation described below will help us to understand fire stagnation. Each one of the six stagnations (see Box 4.1) is identifiable by specific signs and symptoms (Wiseman & Feng 1998).

The Theory of Similar Transformation

According to Liu Wan-su, a great master of internal medicine from the Jin-Yuan dynasties, the host or ruling qi of the organism is yang in nature, and therefore warm. As explained by Flaws, physiologically

BOX 4.1	*The six stagnations and their symptoms*					
	Qi depression	**Blood depression**	**Damp depression**	**Phlegm depression**	**Food depression**	**Fire depression**
	Pain in the chest, rough sunken pulse	Loss of power in the lower limbs, bloody stool, sunken, scallion pulse	General heaviness/ pain, pain in the joints associated with damp weather, sunken pulse	Panting with physical exertion, slippery sunken pulse	Belching of sour gas, abdominal distension, no desire to drink or eat	Visual distortion, oppression and vexation, reddish urine, rapid, sunken pulse

Source: Wiseman & Feng (1998).

this means that 'any evil qi accumulating in the body, whether externally invading or internally engendered will tend to become warm over time because the basic host or ruling qi of the body is hot' (Flaws 1997, p. 52). For this reason, even if a disease was initially caused by cold, or is originally yin in nature, there is a tendency for this disease to transform into a hot pathology if the host yang qi is sufficiently strong (Flaws 1997).

When qi becomes stagnant and depressed, it backs up and accumulates, and may transform into pathological heat or fire because qi is yang in nature. Even though the other four depressions – blood, dampness, phlegm, and food – are originally yin, they obstruct the free flow of qi. The qi tends to become stuck behind or entangled with these yin accumulations, and these four yin depressions also tend to become hot stagnations: dampness tends to become damp heat, stagnant food tends to become complicated by heat, phlegm tends to transform into phlegm heat (or fire), and static blood can become heat stasis (Flaws 1997). In the subsequent sections detailing the evolution of depression patterns, the clinical relevance of the six stagnations, especially qi stagnation, heat transformation, and dampness accumulation, will become clear.

Liver Qi Stagnation: Ramifications and Complications

As explained previously, the liver plays a pivotal role in the precipitation of depressive episodes. When confronted by continuous and prolonged psychosocial or emotional stress, the liver's function of spreading the qi is impaired; the liver cannot maintain its free and unobstructed flow and the qi stagnates. The term 'liver depression qi stagnation' usually refers to qi stagnation due to affect damage

(damage by the emotions), while qi stagnation alone may be due to other causes (Wiseman & Feng 1998). When the qi becomes stagnant due to liver depression, one or more of the following mechanisms are set in motion. Stagnant qi may:

- accumulate along the pathway of the liver channel and its paired channel the gall bladder

- transform into heat

- counterflow sideways or upwards

- result in blood stasis

- result in dampness and phlegm accumulation.

Accumulation

When the qi backs up and accumulates, it may create fullness and distension in the areas traversed by the channels and vessels associated with the liver. The liver channel is connected with the anterior aspect of the legs and thighs, the pelvic region, the abdominal area, the rib cage, the chest, the throat, gums, eyes, and vertex of the head. The clinical symptoms of qi accumulation are oppression in the chest, belching, rib cage, and abdominal distension; additionally, distending pain and the intermittent appearance of a lump are sometimes observed. In addition, functional changes associated with the accumulation of qi along these areas include painful menstrual periods, digestive disturbance, difficulty in breathing, and a feeling of constriction in the throat. The liver connects with the pericardium channel which traverses the anterior aspect of the arms, the upper abdomen, and chest. In fact, the liver and pericardium are considered to be an extension that links the upper and lower regions of the body. The liver and pericardium are known as the *foot jueyin* and *arm jueyin* channels respectively.

Heat Transformation

As mentioned above, qi is yang and therefore, when it accumulates and stagnates, it tends to become hot, and eventually transforms into pathological heat or fire. Because heat is yang in nature and tends to move upwards, this pathological heat may affect the function of those viscera and bowels that are considered to be above the liver, such as the stomach, heart, and lungs. Alternatively it may manifest in the upper parts of the body, such as the mouth, nose, ears, eyes, and head. Because the *shen*, or spirit, resides in the heart, heat due to liver depression may cause the spirit to be agitated or restless. Heat resulting from liver depression qi stagnation is known as *depressive* or *transformative heat*.

Counterflow

The term qi counterflow means a reversal of the normal movement of qi (Wiseman & Feng 1998); it usually implies the venting of excessive liver qi to the areas of the body where it should not be (Schnyer & Flaws 1998). It is said in Chinese Medicine that anger, which is the corresponding emotion for the liver, makes the qi rise. The liver has an interior–exterior (yin–yang) connection with the gall bladder channel, which traverses the lateral aspect of the legs, the sides of the pelvis, the sides of the chest, the sides of the neck, and the temporal aspect of the head. The surplus of qi generated by accumulation of liver qi will tend to move into the gall bladder channel, and may precipitate neck and shoulder tightness and one-sided headaches.

When liver qi counterflows upwards there may be dizziness, headaches, red facial complexion, tinnitus, pain and fullness in the chest and the rib side. If the stomach is affected, there may be belching, burping, acid regurgitation, nausea and vomiting. If it affects the lungs, there may be coughing and wheezing; if the heart is affected there may be insomnia, irritability, and restlessness. If liver qi counterflows horizontally, it may affect the spleen and cause lack of appetite, abdominal distension, and diarrhea.

Accumulation, heat transformation, and counterflow are part of a continuum that is not always so clearly delineated in clinical practice. In Chapter 5, we will provide guidelines to differentiate the treatment principles needed to treat each of these conditions successfully.

Blood Stasis

In addition to regulating the smooth flow of qi (coursing and discharge), the liver stores the blood. In Chinese Medicine it is said that the qi moves the blood and the blood nourishes the qi. When qi fails to move the blood, qi stagnation may cause, and be further exacerbated by, blood stasis (Wiseman & Feng 1998). Long-term or severe qi stagnation may result in blood stasis, and blood stasis due to any other cause may in turn aggravate qi stagnation (Schnyer & Flaws 1998). The simultaneous occurrence of qi stagnation and blood stasis is commonly encountered in clinical practice; it generally involves concomitant symptoms of qi stagnation, such as abdominal distension, and chest oppression with symptoms of blood stasis, such as menstrual pain and clots in the menstruate.

Blood is needed to moisten the liver in order for it to perform smoothly its functions of coursing and discharge. Blood vacuity and, by extension, yin vacuity can create or exacerbate both qi stagnation and blood stasis.

Dampness and Phlegm Accumulation

The qi moves and transforms the body fluids; therefore, prolonged qi stagnation may result in dampness accumulation, and dampness may lead to phlegm. Phlegm can then lodge in the viscera and bowels, the channels and network vessels, or in the body's orifices, further exacerbating the obstruction of qi and affecting the functions of those viscera, channels, and orifices (Schnyer & Flaws 1998). Dampness accumulation and phlegm obstruction arising for any other reason may also precipitate and exacerbate liver qi stagnation.

Yin Fire

Yin fire is a complex theory developed by another great master of internal medicine, Li Dong-yuan, who is known as founder of the school of thought known as *Supplementing Earth* (spleen) and author of the *Pi Wei Lun* (Treatise of the Spleen and Stomach). Yin fire refers to heat that stems from the spleen and that is associated with dampness; it is heat that arises from the yin or lower part of the body. It is a type of pathological (yin) heat versus the healthy (yang) heat. Yin fire (*yin huo*) should not be confused with vacuity heat (*xu re*); vacuity heat is a type of yin fire, but yin fire is a larger and more complex category which includes vacuity heat (Flaws 1997). Vacuity heat is due to insufficiency of yin; yin fire is due, in part, to an accumulation of a yin substance which has transformed into heat.

There are five basic mechanisms associated with the production of yin fire: spleen vacuity, damp heat, liver stagnation, blood (yin) vacuity, stirring of ministerial fire. These five mechanisms are interdependent, and they mutually engender and promote one another (Flaws 1997).

Spleen Vacuity

Spleen vacuity is considered the root of yin fire. If the spleen becomes vacuous and weak, and loses its ability to control the movement and transformation of body fluids, these fluids tend to gather and accumulate, eventually transforming into dampness.

Damp Heat

The dampness generated by spleen vacuity will tend to pour downwards; dampness accumulation over a long period of time may eventually become damp heat. Even though this damp heat is located in the lower burner,[1] the heat moves upwards, further disturbing the spleen and damaging the heart and lungs above.

Liver Stagnation

As mentioned above, the liver and spleen have a very close relationship via the control cycle of the five phases. Spleen vacuity may cause or aggravate liver depression qi stagnation. The spleen is responsible for the engenderment and transformation of qi and blood; if spleen vacuity precipitates blood vacuity, insufficient blood will not properly moisten and harmonize the liver. Spleen vacuity is, therefore, directly connected with liver depression; furthermore, since liver depression qi stagnation tends to transform into heat, spleen vacuity is frequently found in conjunction with depressive heat. Liver yang is part of the *life gate fire*,[2] or *ministerial fire*, the basic fire of life (i.e. kidney yang). Therefore, depressive heat that originates in the liver causes stirring of ministerial fire below, additionally affecting the spleen, stomach, lungs, and heart above.

Blood (Yin) Vacuity

When the spleen becomes vacuous and weak, it loses its ability to engender and transform the blood, creating blood vacuity. Blood vacuity may eventually affect kidney yin because blood and essence share a common source, just as the liver and the kidneys share a common source. Liver blood–kidney yin vacuity precipitates vacuity heat. Vacuity heat originates in the lower burner or yin part of the body; therefore it is also considered a type of yin fire. This vacuity heat counterflows upwards and affects the liver, spleen, stomach, lungs, and heart.

Stirring of Ministerial Fire

Ministerial fire is the fire in the body that inhabits the life gate (*ming men*), liver, gall bladder, and triple heater, and it is thought to originate from and be inseparable from kidney yang. Ministerial fire is the

---

[1]The lower burner refers to the part of the triple burner that includes the kidney, bladder, large intestine, and small intestine, in their function of drawing fluids to be discharged in the form of urine (Wiseman & Feng 1998). The triple burner is one of the six bowels comprising the upper, middle, and lower burners; it is a way of describing the combined function of different viscera and bowels by grouping them and dividing the body into three sections. It is referred to as the 'waterways', meaning that the main functions of the triple burner are the processing of fluids by the transformation of qi and ensuring free flow through the waterways (Wiseman & Feng 1988).
[2]The life gate is a 'physiological entity of disputed morphological identity' (Wiseman & Feng 1998). Some consider the life gate to be the space between the kidneys; others consider it to be contained in both kidneys. The life gate is referred to as the root of original qi and the house of fire and water, the stirring qi between the kidneys, the fire of the true yang for the whole body.

complementary opposite to the *sovereign fire*, or fire of the heart. Stirring of ministerial fire is due to overactivity and overstimulation, as well as to excessive sexual activity. It is a condition in which the ministerial fire below becomes hyperactive and agitated, and it flames upwards (Wiseman & Feng 1998), harassing and damaging the viscera and bowels above it.

Yin fire is an invaluable theory for understanding the evolution of depression patterns and is the most common complex pattern combinations encountered in depressed patients. It is extremely common to encounter spleen vacuity, dampness, and phlegm accumulation, concomitant with liver depression transforming into heat. On the one hand the phlegm and dampness cause psychomotor retardation symptoms, lack of interest, apathy, and lethargy; on the other, the heat from qi stagnation causes agitation, anxiety, and in most cases insomnia. Recall that following the classical classification of psychiatric disorders according to Chinese Medicine (CM), depression falls within the *withdrawal* category; withdrawal is precipitated by either qi and/or yang vacuity, or by the yang qi not flowing freely due to liver depression and phlegm obstruction. Nevertheless, major depressive episodes are rarely, if ever, devoid of some degree of agitation and heat.

In our experience, having evaluated dozens of clients presenting with clinical depression, major depressive episodes are most often characterized by a combination of spleen–kidney dual vacuity, dampness and phlegm accumulation, and depressive heat from liver qi stagnation. The degree of severity and variety of manifestations is dependent on the person's constitution and lifestyle, as well as the etiology of the depressive episode. Of course there are a few cases of depression primarily due to vacuity, especially spleen qi–heart blood vacuity, and there are a few cases that manifest primarily with repletion signs, such as liver depression and phlegm obstruction.

Constitutional tendencies towards either yin or yang vacuity precipitate or aggravate liver depression in specific ways. On one hand, as yin and blood develop from the same source, blood vacuity can lead to yin vacuity; because yin blood is what nourishes the liver and facilitates its functions of coursing and discharge, yin vacuity may also aggravate liver depression. When yin becomes vacuous, it may lead to yang becoming effulgent, which in turn generates internal heat. On the other hand, spleen qi vacuity may eventually affect the kidney and result in spleen qi–kidney yang vacuity. It is kidney yang, the life gate fire or ministerial fire, which promotes the liver function of maintaining free flow; therefore, spleen qi–kidney yang vacuity is rarely seen in people experiencing depression without concomitant liver depression qi stagnation. Additionally, spleen qi–kidney yang vacuity tends to aggravate liver depression qi stagnation (Schnyer & Flaws 1998).

With the preceding as a background, we now discuss how these mechanisms precipitate the patterns seen in depression. Qi stagnation, heat transformation, spleen and kidney vacuity, and dampness and phlegm accumulation can combine to produce the complex patterns characteristic of major depressive episodes.

EVOLUTION OF PATTERNS OF DEPRESSION

The patterns encountered in people experiencing depression are generally composed of elements of both vacuity and repletion. As explained above, patterns of depression develop as a result of the interaction of four main disease mechanisms: (1) those that evolve from liver depression qi stagnation, (2) those that directly affect the heart's function of housing the *shen* or spirit, (3) those that derive from vacuity of either qi–yang or blood–yin, and (4) those that derive from repletion – the accumulation of dampness and phlegm, or hyperactivity of yang. Depression patterns are complex, formed by several different 'basic patterns' of both vacuity and repletion.

Repletion Disease Mechanisms

Damage by the emotions in the form of emotional stress and frustration compromises the liver's ability for coursing and discharge; liver depression qi stagnation, if severe or enduring over a prolonged period of time, may transform into heat and eventually into fire. Depressive heat counterflows upwards, agitating the heart and spirit. Liver depression may eventually lead to blood stasis, to food stagnation, or may precipitate and aggravate spleen vacuity. If the spleen is vacuous and weak, it may not be able to transform and transport fluids, thus leading to dampness accumulation and eventually to phlegm. Phlegm may be drafted upwards by counterflowing qi, misting the heart and causing confusion and disorientation. It may also become bound in the chest and affect both the heart and the lung, or it may combine with depressive heat or fire, both agitating and misting the heart (Fig. 4.1).

Vacuity Disease Mechanisms

By the same token, following the progression of liver depression qi stagnation, an overactivity in the liver may cause or further

FIGURE 4.1   *Evolution of depression patterns: repletion*

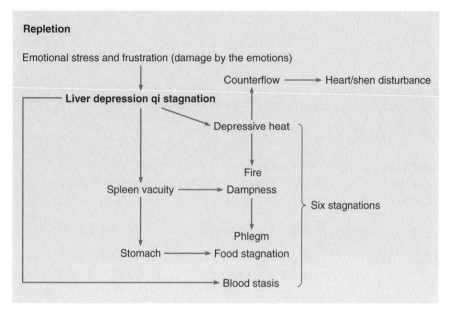

Damage by the emotions precipitates liver depression qi stagnation which, in turn, may transform into heat or fire and counterflow, affecting the heart and disturbing the shen. It may also attack and weaken the spleen, rendering it incapable of transforming dampness, allowing phlegm to accumulate, or damaging the stomach and leading to food stagnation. Enduring or severe liver depression may also result in blood stasis. The development of the six stagnations – heat, fire, dampness, phlegm, food, and blood – is also shown.

exacerbate a predisposition to spleen vacuity. If the spleen becomes vacuous and weak, it will not only become incapable of transforming and transporting body fluids (a function of spleen qi), but will also fail to generate sufficient blood (and qi). This may lead to heart qi and heart blood vacuity, rendering the heart unable to store the spirit. This blood vacuity may precipitate kidney yin vacuity since the essence and the blood share a common source, as do the liver and kidney. Furthermore, depressive heat and fire may further damage the blood and yin, further exacerbating yin vacuity and giving rise to a hyperactivity of yang or fire effulgence. If spleen vacuity endures over a prolonged period of time, it may eventually progress into kidney qi and yang vacuity (Fig. 4.2).

Patterns of both vacuity and repletion can affect the heart's ability to house the *shen* or spirit (i.e. *shen disturbance*), as depicted in Figure 4.3. Specifically, repletion patterns that affect the *shen* may develop from either liver depression qi stagnation or dampness and phlegm accumulation (due to spleen vacuity). Those that develop from liver depression include stagnation of heart and lung qi,

FIGURE 4.2   *Evolution of depression patterns: vacuity*

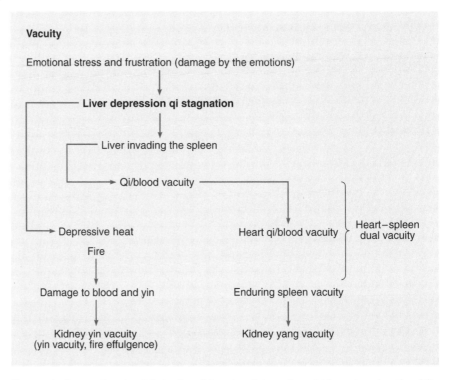

Damage by the emotions precipitates liver depression qi stagnation, which compromises the ability of the spleen to generate qi and blood. Qi and blood vacuity may lead to heart qi or heart blood vacuity and, if severe or prolonged, to kidney vacuity as well. If liver depression transforms into heat or fire, it may damage blood and yin, and may lead to yin vacuity and vacuity heat.

depressive heat affecting the heart, and heart fire. Patterns that stem from dampness and phlegm accumulation include phlegm obstruction and stagnation, phlegm confounding the orifices of the heart, and phlegm fire harassing the heart. In turn, vacuity patterns affecting the *shen* generally derive from spleen qi–kidney yang vacuity or from liver blood–kidney yin vacuity. Heart blood and heart qi vacuity stem from spleen qi–kidney yang vacuity. Heart yin vacuity and vacuity heat generally stem from liver blood–kidney yin vacuity.

Again, depending on predisposing factors and the constellation of signs and symptoms, the nature of the depressive episode will vary greatly among individuals. It is still to be determined by further research, but the theory would predict that chronic or recurrent depressions, dysthymia, and nonspecified depressive disorder are characterized by significant and long-standing phlegm obstruction and blood stasis and/or by extreme insufficiency of qi and blood, or both.

| FIGURE 4.3 | *The evolution of vacuity and repletion patterns that result in shen disturbance* |

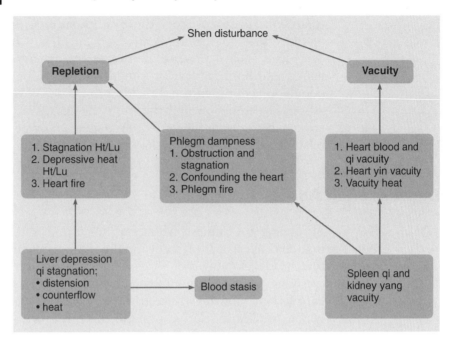

This figure shows the evolution of patterns that affect the heart's function of housing the shen, due to either vacuity or repletion. On the left-hand side it is shown how shen disturbance due to repletion manifests as one of three patterns stemming originally from liver depression. On the right-hand side it is shown how three patterns stemming from spleen qi and kidney yang vacuity manifest as shen disturbance due to vacuity. In the middle, the relationship between spleen vacuity, liver depression, and dampness and phlegm is illustrated by three patterns that develop as a combination of vacuity and repletion disease mechanisms. Ht, heart; Lu, lung.

DEPRESSION AND THE LIFE CYCLE

According to Chinese Medicine, the disease mechanisms that are set into motion during depressive episodes are determined in part by the stage of the life cycle in which we find ourselves. The tendency to develop liver depression may be exacerbated by one's age or occupation; the constitutional tendency towards vacuity or repletion patterns may be influenced by diet and lifestyle choices. The following discussion represents an extension of the framework that we have used to date in our research studies. Thus, while the following section may be regarded as an untested extension of our approach, these addendums derive directly from eight principles theory and therefore should be consistent with our current approach. These extensions of our framework involve how depression appears in adolescence, how depression develops in women in relationship to pregnancy and menopause, and how aging may affect the predisposition to depression. This augmented framework can be used as the basis for the development of a treatment protocol for these populations, given appropriate modifications to the applications detailed in Chapter 5. We have developed such a protocol for research in depression during pregnancy, and hope to develop similar protocols for use with the other populations in the future. In addition, we will cover in this section an aspect of depression and the life cycle that is a part of the current approach we use in our research: namely, how depression in women relates to the menstrual cycle.

Depression in Adolescence

According to Chinese Medicine, the rapid and dramatic changes that characterize adolescence make it a particularly vulnerable time for the development of disease mechanisms related to depressive episodes. Sexual development is a function of exuberance of the life gate fire or ministerial fire (the *ming men* or yang of the kidney), which implies a relative repletion of yang qi. This exuberance of yang necessary for growth and development acts as a natural fuel which quickly transforms any accumulation into heat or fire. The stirring up of ministerial fire agitates the liver, stomach, spleen, heart, and lungs. In addition, common frustrations characteristic of adolescence render the liver incapable of maintaining the smooth flow of qi. As mentioned above, liver repletion weakens the spleen's ability to generate qi and blood, and to transform dampness; this weakness is frequently exacerbated by indulging in a poor diet, and by abusing drugs or alcohol.

Depression in a Woman's Life

Depression is twice as common in women as in men (Kessler et al 1994); this fact can be explained, in part, by the Chinese Medicine view of the relationship between liver depression and the menstrual cycle. This is not to say that the higher incidence of depression in women is merely due to hormonal imbalances. Depression is the result of complex interactions between diverse factors, many of which are not yet fully understood; some of these factors can be explained biologically, many others cannot (see Ch. 2).

Because our research protocol excluded women during pregnancy, and did not aim at addressing specifically postpartum depression, we will first review the mechanism of depression in relationship to menstruation and menopause. In subsequent sections, we will review considerations for treating depression in conditions that extend beyond our research protocol, including depression during pregnancy and postpartum depression.

The Menstrual Cycle

According to Chinese Medicine, the heart, spleen, and kidney play important roles in the *creation* of blood. The spleen transforms food and liquids into nourishment, and sends the finest essence of food extracted through the process of digestion up for the heart to transform it into blood, while the kidney also sends some essence to the heart. It is said in Chinese Medicine that it is in the heart that the blood becomes red and is finally created (Schnyer & Flaws 1998).

Insufficient creation of blood may be due to: (1) an inability of the spleen to extract the finest essence of food and send it to the heart, (2) a lack of sufficient essence coming from the kidney, or (3) the inability of the heart to complete the creation of blood and its distribution to the whole body. It is only after the blood has nourished and moistened the viscera and bowels, the channels and vessels, and the rest of the tissues of the body, that the remaining surplus accumulates in the uterus to be discharged as menstrual blood. In addition, three viscera *control* the movement and distribution of blood: the heart, the liver, and the spleen. Specifically, what moves the blood is the heart qi, which in turn originates primarily from the qi of the spleen. In addition, the spleen also restrains and controls the blood within its pathways, while the liver qi stores the blood by regulating the amount of blood in circulation at any given time. The flow and rhythm of the menstrual cycle depend upon the heart and spleen to provide the motivating force or qi for the blood to move, and upon the liver's ability to maintain the free and uninterrupted movement of qi, and therefore, blood. For menstruation to take place, there must be sufficient blood, and the qi and blood must be able to move freely and without interruption (Schnyer & Flaws 1998).

The Phases of the Menstrual Cycle According to Chinese Medicine

A predisposition to depression and the prevalence of some depressive symptoms may vary according to the phases of the menstrual cycle. Chinese Medicine divides the menstrual cycle into four phases.

End of Menstruation

At the end of menstruation, the body is left relatively empty of blood, a yin substance. If there is an underlying vacuity of yin, the body may have difficulty in replenishing the blood that has been lost. Symptoms due to blood or yin vacuity may become exacerbated at this time. In addition, the yin may become unable to restrain yang, and heat and fire may flare upward and agitate the spirit. The focus of the treatment strategy should emphasize replenishing and nourishing the yin and blood and, if necessary, clear heat and drain fire.

Ovulation

The time around ovulation is characterized by the transformation of yin into yang. It is necessary to have sufficient yin to transform into yang, and to have enough yang for this transformation to take place. If the body has not been able to replenish the yin and blood during the previous phase, or if the qi and blood are not flowing freely, this transformation will also be impeded. On the other hand, if yin has been replenished successfully during phase one, the growth of yang may exacerbate underlying heat or fire, or add heat to liver depression, transforming qi stagnation into depressive heat. This yang heat may flare upwards and agitate the spirit. The focus of the intervention should be to facilitate the movement of qi and blood, and to clear heat or drain fire.

Premenstruum

Premenstrually, the qi must flow freely and in the right direction, and the yang must stay strong for a sufficient length of time. Because the qi and blood continue to focus and accumulate inward and downward towards the uterus, the body is usually at its hottest, because qi is yang and yang is hot. If the qi and blood are not flowing freely due to liver depression, or if qi accumulation transforms into heat or fire and flares upwards, or if the yang is not strong enough to move the qi and blood downwards, depressive symptoms tend to exacerbate premenstrually. Additionally, the liver's function of coursing and discharge depends on the nourishment of the liver by the blood; in a woman with blood vacuity, what little blood she has will tend to accumulate in her uterus, and leave the rest of her body more empty. This may exacerbate liver depression on the one hand, and heart blood and yin vacuity on the other, aggravating the corresponding symptoms of depression. As above, the treatment of depression should emphasize coursing the liver, rectifying the qi, and clearing heat.

Menstruation

During the menstrual period itself, with the discharge of blood and the release of qi that goes along with it, there is generally a reduction in the signs and symptoms of depression associated with liver depression qi stagnation. Treatment principles should focus on supporting this movement of qi and the discharge of blood. Although theoretically, in both phases three and four, symptoms may be exacerbated by insufficiency of qi and yang, in treating depression one should focus on coursing the liver, rectifying qi, and clearing heat from the time of ovulation until the onset of the menstrual period.

In our protocol, we divide the treatment of depression in women during their menstruating years into two general phases. In the first half of the cycle, from the end of menstruation to before ovulation, we emphasize addressing the repletion components of the pattern by rectifying qi, clearing heat, draining fire, and eliminating dampness or transforming phlegm, as necessary. In the second half of the cycle, from ovulation through the onset of menstruation, we focus on addressing primarily the vacuity components of the complex pattern, by boosting qi, nourishing blood, enriching yin and fortifying the spleen, kidney (and lung), as necessary. During menstruation itself, we balance out our strategy, depending on the presentation. Please refer to the section on Strategies and Techniques in Chapter 5 for examples of point selection.

Depression and Menopause

According to Chinese Medicine, blood is considered to be the outward manifestation of essence. As explained above, essence can be *inherited* or *acquired*. Inherited essence is used up through the process of living and cannot be supplemented. Acquired essence is the surplus of qi (energy) and blood (nourishment) that is produced for daily functioning through the process of digestion, performed by the spleen. With age, digestion becomes less efficient and a woman's body no longer produces a surplus of blood to maintain a monthly period without this loss of blood becoming draining. In a sense, by using more qi and blood that can be produced effectively through digestion, one begins to 'borrow' from the original reservoir – the inherited essence that is stored in the kidney. Therefore, according to Chinese Medicine, menopause is viewed as a homeostatic mechanism that, in fact, slows down the process of aging. Menopause is characterized by a cessation of menstruation precisely because its purpose is to preserve the essence (Wolfe 1998).

The uterus (*bao gong*) is considered an extraordinary organ, connected to the kidney via the *bao luo*, and to the heart via *bao mai* (uterine network vessels). 'The uterine vessels home to the heart and net to the uterus' (Wiseman & Feng 1998, p. 643). The uterus is related to the kidney essence, the chong and ren channels, and the heart, liver, and spleen. During menstruating years, the heart sends blood down to collect in the uterus via the *bao mai*; gradually, as menopause approaches, the heart stops doing this, and menstruation becomes irregular. This illustrates one of the mechanisms through which the heart and kidney are intimately related, and emphasizes the connection between the spirit and the essence, the psyche and the soma, the body and the mind. When menstruation finally stops and the heart no longer sends blood downward to the uterus, the flow in the *bao mai* reverses itself, and the essence is sent up to the heart to nourish the woman's spirit. As Flaws (1992) summarizes in his book *My Sister the Moon*, 'instead of preparing the uterus for the growth of a physical addition to the community of humankind, the blood focuses on the heart to nourish the woman's spirit' (p. 315).

The factors that contribute to an increased predisposition to experiencing depression during a transition into menopause depend on the ability of the liver to maintain the free flow of qi, on the capacity of the spleen to generate sufficient qi and blood, and on the condition of the kidney essence.

Depression during Pregnancy

The disease mechanisms that can determine a woman's risk for depression during pregnancy develop in basically the same way as they do for depressive episodes in general; therefore, they can be explained by evaluating the vacuity and repletion elements of the four features mentioned above.

The process of pregnancy per se places specific demands upon the viscera and bowels that can affect the free and smooth flow of qi throughout the body, the engenderment and transformation of qi and blood, and the movement and transformation of body fluids. The viscera most affected include the liver, the kidney, and the spleen. These factors may potentially increase a woman's predisposition to experience a depressive episode during pregnancy.

During the first trimester of pregnancy, when menstruation ceases, blood and qi back up in the liver; the liver becomes replete and loses its ability for coursing and discharging, which creates or exacerbates a predisposition to liver qi stagnation. In addition, the liver stores the blood and it is closely related to *chong mai*, the 'sea of blood', one of the eight extraordinary vessels (see Channels and Network Vessels in Ch. 3). Among other functions, this channel sends blood down to the uterus and it continues to do so after conception. As the fetus cannot yet make full use of all the blood accumulating in the uterus, it blocks the *uterine gate*, further aggravating liver qi stagnation (Flaws 1992). As explained above, if prolonged, liver depression may transform into heat or fire, and it can precipitate or aggravate blood stasis.

Throughout pregnancy there is an increased demand for qi and blood to nourish and promote the development of the fetus; this may weaken the spleen by placing an increased demand on its functions, which may result in insufficiency of qi and blood, or cause dampness to accumulate, thus leading to phlegm (Flaws 1992).

After conception it is the kidney that nourishes the fetus with essence. Blood and essence share a common source; because the kidney is also the source of yin, when so much blood and essence are focused on nourishing the fetus, the rest of the body may suffer an insufficiency of yin. This vacuity of yin may lead to yang becoming replete, and yang repletion may counterflow upwards, causing agitation and restlessness. If the yin of the kidney is insufficient, it may be unable both to nourish the fetus and to moisten and relax the liver.

The heart in turn depends on sufficient blood to perform properly its function of housing the spirit, maintaining awareness, and integrating our being. An insufficiency of blood due to spleen qi vacuity may in turn precipitate or aggravate a disturbance of *shen* due to heart blood vacuity. The section on Strategies and Techniques in Chapter 5 discusses adapting this protocol to the treatment of depression during pregnancy.

Postpartum Depression

The process of labor and delivery, in conjunction with specific features of the postpartum period, may lead to disease mechanisms that can precipitate depression. According to Chinese Medicine there are two main disease mechanisms that characterize the onset of depression during the postpartum period. Vacuity patterns may develop from excessive blood loss (and fluid loss through profuse perspiration) and excessive use of qi through exertion during labor. Excessive loss of blood during delivery may leave the heart qi and blood vacuous and weak. Because the blood nourishes and secures the spirit, blood vacuity may lead the *shen* to become unsettled, resulting in anxiety and restlessness. A prolonged and difficult labor resulting in extreme exertion can lead to qi vacuity of both the kidney and the spleen; this gives rise to fatigue and to what is known in Chinese Medicine as *lassitude of spirit* (lack of mental vigor and physical strength). In addition, because the blood nourishes the liver and allows it to maintain the smooth movement of qi and blood, blood vacuity may cause or exacerbate qi stagnation (Flaws 1997).

Repletion patterns primarily result from or become exacerbated by liver depression qi stagnation. For many women, the postpartum phase is characterized by a mixture of awe and elation on the one hand, and unforeseen psychosocial stressors on the other; the natural stress of caring for a newborn child may further aggravate a predisposition to liver depression qi stagnation.

If for some reason stagnant blood is retained after delivery, or the postpartum lochia is not expelled properly, blood stasis may exacerbate qi stagnation. Blood stasis and stagnation can counterflow upwards, penetrating and disturbing the heart. In addition, heart blood and spleen qi vacuity may aggravate blood stasis. When blood loss results in heart blood vacuity, the blood vessels are not well nourished and are less capable of moving and transporting the blood. When exertion results in qi vacuity, there is less qi available to move and transport the blood (Flaws 1997).

Liver depression can result in spleen vacuity and an accumulation of dampness and phlegm. In addition, because of the hard work of labor and delivery, and the tremendous physical demand to produce enough nutritious breast milk for a newborn, postpartum women crave rich foods, which unfortunately are also very difficult to digest. If the spleen is already weak and possibly affected by liver depression counterflow, overeating rich foods may also contribute to the production of dampness and phlegm. Enduring or severe liver depression may transform into depressive heat. This heat may stew and congeal the water fluids, also resulting in phlegm. Phlegm may obstruct the orifices of the heart, and obscure the functions of the *shen* or spirit, or it may combine with depressive heat and develop into phlegm fire. Special considerations for treating depression during pregnancy and contraindications can be found in Strategies and Techniques in Chapter 5.

Depression and Aging

According to Chinese Medicine, aging is a decline in the production and free flow of qi and blood. Traditionally, problems related to aging have been addressed in Chinese Medicine by emphasizing supplementation of qi, blood, yang, and/or yin. However, Yan De-Xin (1995), a leading Chinese physician who has revolutionized the field of TCM geriatrics, affirms that the chief mechanism of aging is the loss of regulation and harmony of qi and blood (i.e. stagnation; De-Xin 1995).

In addition, prolonged or severe qi stagnation results in blood stasis. For these two reasons, in the elderly the vacuity disease mechanisms that characterize depression are likely to be complicated by not only qi stagnation but also by blood stasis.

Five main disease mechanisms help us to understand the progression and development of depression in the elderly:

1. A decline of essence that depends on the kidney, and which in turn affects the kidney's function of providing the foundation for both yin and yang

2. A weakening of the spleen's ability to transform food into nourishment, which affects both the production and the movement of qi and blood

3. An aggravation of liver depression qi stagnation in turn due to qi and/or yang vacuity, and vacuity of blood and/or yin

4. The inability of the heart to house the *shen* or spirit due to blood and yin vacuity

5. A weakness of the *shen* itself due to qi vacuity.

Decline of Essence

As explained above, the kidney stores the essence; there are two types of essence – inherited and acquired. Because inherited essence is finite, it cannot be replaced or augmented; it is spent through the process of living. The rate at which we grow older is dependent upon our constitutional endowment of this essence and upon how well we take care of it. Stress, overwork, excessive sexual activity, and drug and alcohol use all contribute to the depletion of our inherited essence.

Weakness of Spleen Function

Our acquired essence, on the other hand, is derived from food and drink, and is dependent upon the spleen's function of transforming food into qi and blood. Acquired essence helps to enhance and support our inherited essence: if one eats well and the process of digestion is effective, and if one does not spend more qi and blood than are created each day, then during sleep the surplus of qi and blood is transformed into essence. Around the age of 35 years the spleen becomes weak and its ability to transform food into nourishment begins to decline. The reserves of inherited essence are tapped and eventually, because of the interdependence of the spleen and the kidney, the kidney also becomes weak. The production of qi and blood becomes progressively more scanty (Schnyer & Flaws 1998).

Aggravation of Liver Depression Qi Stagnation

The free movement of qi can take place effectively only if there is sufficient qi being created to propel it. Similarly, there must be enough blood to moisten and nourish the liver to maintain its function of regulating the smooth flow of qi. Symptoms of liver depression tend to increase when there is less qi or less blood available. In addition, the functions of the liver depend on the yang of the kidney, which provides the foundation for the production and movement of qi. In sum, liver depression can be aggravated by qi and yang vacuity on the one hand, and yin and blood vacuity on the other.

Inability of the Heart to House the Shen

The blood provides the material foundation for the *shen* or spirit; without enough blood, the heart loses its ability to house or anchor the *shen*. When there is a decline of blood, the *shen* becomes unquiet and restless; symptoms of heart blood and yin vacuity, such as insomnia, anxiety, and fidgetiness tend to increase.

Weakness of Shen

Because the *shen* or spirit is understood as the accumulation of qi and blood in the heart, a decline in the production of qi would make the *shen* weaker, less bright, and less clear.

RELATIONSHIP BETWEEN THE THEORETICAL FRAMEWORK AND THE APPLICATION OF THE TREATMENT APPROACH

Chapters 3 and 4 have provided the background for understanding the causes of and progression of depressive symptoms from the perspective of Chinese Medicine. Chapter 5 details how to differentiate various patterns on the basis of signs and symptoms, many of which have been described in the previous two chapters. Chapter 5 further describes how to develop appropriate treatment principles and how to select acupuncture points to design the correct treatments to address those principles.

5 Application of Traditional Chinese Medicine in the Diagnosis and Treatment of Depression

THE TREATMENT OF PATTERNS OF DISHARMONY INVOLVED IN DEPRESSION

Chapters 3, 4 and 5 are meant to be read as a unit; Chapters 3 and 4 present the essential background for the application of the framework outlined in Chapter 5. The absence of understanding of the disease mechanisms that precipitate the patterns and of the rationale for point selection will provide, at best, a mechanical cook-book approach to treatment that will fail to address the complexity of depression as experienced by most people. We strongly recommend reading these three chapters sequentially.

Based on the proposed framework, depressive episodes are generally characterized by the combination of various patterns. To determine the disease mechanisms relevant to the different pattern combinations, one needs to evaluate to what extent the following four features are present in each person:

- Qi stagnation, stemming from the liver's inability to perform its function of coursing and discharge

- Shen disturbance, arising from the heart's inability to perform its function of housing the spirit (*shen*) due to either *vacuity* or *repletion*

- Yin features including (a) qi and yang *vacuity* (yang) and/or (b) *repletion* of dampness and phlegm (yin)

■ Yang features including (a) yin and blood *vacuity* (yin) and/or (b) repletion of heat or fire (yang).

In addition, one needs to identify which specific viscera and bowels are involved. Generally, a person experiencing depression does not fit only one pattern, and similarly does not present with an imbalance in only one viscus or bowel. It is common clinically to encounter a complex combination of patterns which includes elements of these four features. The particular complex pattern combination will determine the treatment principles and the individually tailored treatment plan. For example, a person might present with: (1) stagnant liver qi, transforming into heat (depressive heat), and (2) heart blood vacuity, and (3) spleen qi vacuity. The pattern then will be: liver depression transforms heat, heart–spleen dual vacuity. The treatment principles will be: course the liver and rectify the qi, clear heat and resolve depression, fortify the spleen and nourish the heart, boost the qi and supplement the blood.

Traditionally, the disease mechanisms are evaluated first, then the patterns and combination of patterns are determined, then the treatment principles are outlined, and finally a treatment plan is designed. Some of the patterns emerging from the four features mentioned above, and some pattern combinations, are particularly relevant in depression, while others are not. To facilitate pattern differentiation and to clarify the disease mechanisms underlying depression, the patterns that become the building blocks for more complex patterns will first be reviewed. Within the description of each pattern, the natural progression of depression patterns will be described, and then common pattern combinations may be listed under 'special considerations' for that pattern. Then the 12 most commonly encountered basic and combined patterns that precipitate depression will be listed.

At the end of this chapter there is a summary (Tables 5.1A, B & C) that presents this information in condensed form for easy reference.

The main basic patterns involved in major depression are:

1. **Qi stagnation**

   a. Liver depression qi stagnation
   b. Liver depression transforms heat
   c. Qi stagnation affecting the heart and lung
   d. Blood stasis and stagnation

2. **Shen disturbance: vacuity**

   a. Heart blood vacuity
   b. Heart qi vacuity
   c. Heart yin vacuity
   d. Heart fire flaming upward (heart yin vacuity with vacuity heat)

3. **Shen disturbance: repletion**

   a. Qi stagnation affecting the heart and lung
   b. Depressive heat affecting the heart or lung
   c. Exuberant heart fire
   d. Phlegm confounding the heart (orifices)
   e. Phlegm (heat) fire harassing the heart

4. **Qi/yang vacuity**

   a. Spleen/lung qi vacuity
   b. Spleen yang vacuity
   c. Kidney qi vacuity
   d. Kidney yang vacuity

5. **Dampness and phlegm**

   a. Spleen vacuity, dampness accumulation
   b. Phlegm confounding the heart (orifices)
   c. Heart vacuity, gall bladder timidity
   d. Phlegm dampness obstruction and stagnation
   e. Phlegm fire harassing the heart

6. **Blood/yin vacuity**

   a. Heart blood vacuity
   b. Liver blood vacuity
   c. Liver yin vacuity
   d. Kidney yin vacuity
   e. Lung yin vacuity

7. **Yang repletion and vacuity heat**

   a. Liver depression transforms heat
   b. Hyperactivity of liver yang
   c. Liver fire flaming upward
   d. Yin vacuity, fire effulgence (vacuity heat)
   e. Spleen vacuity giving rise to fire (yin fire)

THE PATTERNS

Much of the material concerning the specific patterns derives from two comprehensive sources: Finney & Flaws (1996) and Maciocia (1994). Information concerning symptoms specific to depression has been adapted from clinical observation and integrated with the material from these sources to produce the protocol outlined below.

Qi stagnation

Liver depression qi stagnation

Disease causes, disease mechanisms: Emotional stress, anger, and frustration cause the liver to lose its ability to regulate coursing and discharge; there is emotional depression and lack of smooth flow of the qi mechanism. The qi becomes stagnant along the pathway of the liver channel, which traverses the lower abdomen and stomach, and spreads across the chest and sides of the ribs. One may see abdominal and chest oppression, pain along the ribs; if the liver attacks the stomach, the stomach loses its harmony and downbearing; there may be epigastric oppression, belching and burping, possibly nausea and vomiting; if it affects the spleen, there is loss of appetite, abdominal distension, and diarrhea.

Main symptoms: Chest, lateral, costal, breast and abdominal distension and oppression, sighing, dysmenorrhea, irregular menstruation, premenstrual tension, a feeling of a lump in the throat; nausea, vomiting, hiccups, burping, belching, if the liver is invading the stomach.

Symptoms associated with depression: Irritability, mental depression, moodiness, feeling wound-up, alternation of moods, snapping easily, and an intense feeling of frustration.

Pulse: Wiry.

Tongue: Normal or slightly dark, thin coating.

Treatment principles: Course the liver, rectify the qi, and resolve depression.

Main acupuncture points: Lv 3, LI 4.

Additional points: Lv 14, UB 18.

Adjacent points:

- For chest and breast distension and pain: Ren 17 or Sp 21
- For lower abdominal distension or pain: Ren 6, Ren 4, St 28, St 29
- For hypochondriac distension and pain: Lv 14
- For epigastric fullness and distension: Ren 12.

Special considerations: Only in very acute and uncomplicated depressive episodes may liver depression qi stagnation cause depression all by itself. Liver depression qi stagnation usually combines with, and aggravates, pre-existing tendencies towards imbalances in other viscera and bowels. The specific mechanisms triggered by a failure in the functions of coursing and discharge determine the individual's symptoms of depression, the nature and duration of the depressive episode, and the prognosis and outcome of the treatment. However, most major depressive episodes seem to involve liver depression qi stagnation as a significant component. In dysthymia as well as recurrent, chronic, and recalcitrant depression, liver depression qi stagnation seems to precipitate phlegm obstruction and blood stasis, and/or occurs on a background of long-standing constitutional insufficiency.

Qi stagnation

Liver depression transforms heat

Disease causes, disease mechanisms: Extreme or long-term stagnation of liver qi will eventually transform into heat. Because heat is yang in nature, it tends to counterflow or move upwards, negatively affecting the function of organs (stomach, heart, and lungs) and tissues (head, mouth, nose, ears, and eyes) located above the liver. In addition to symptoms of qi stagnation, there will be symptoms of heat. This heat can force the blood to move recklessly, outside its pathways. Because the spirit resides in the heart, upwardly counterflowing depressive heat may disturb the heart spirit, causing it to become restless. (See below under Depressive heat affecting the heart or lung.)

Main symptoms: Insomnia, excessive dreams, chest oppression, agitation, red eyes, red facial complexion, acne, heart palpitations; breast distension but more prominent pain, hypersensitive nipples; bitter taste in the mouth, thirst; early or excessive menstruation, dysfunctional uterine bleeding.

Symptoms associated with depression: Irascibility, easy anger, impetuosity, mental restlessness, aggression, violent outbursts of anger.

Pulse: Wiry and rapid.

Tongue: Dark and red and/or swollen edges, with a thin yellow coat.

Treatment principles: Course the liver and rectify the qi, clear heat, and resolve depression.

Main acupuncture points: UB 18, UB 15, Lv 2 and Lv 3, LI 4, LI 11, P 7, Ht 5.

Additional acupuncture points: Add points to settle the heart and calm the spirit, and/or points to open the chest and stimulate the descending of lung qi.

Special considerations: When enduring or severe liver depression transforms into heat or fire, this heat is known as depressive heat. In addition to anger and frustration, any of the seven emotions may transform into fire, if extreme. Depressive heat may be aggravated by heat accumulating in the stomach due to eating hot, spicy, and greasy fatty foods or drinking alcohol. If, in addition to liver depression qi stagnation, there is dampness and phlegm due to spleen vacuity, the stomach may further lose its ability to digest the food, and food may accumulate. It is not uncommon to find symptoms of food stagnation such as bad breath, nausea, indigestion, thick, slimy tongue fur, and a slippery pulse complicating other patterns. As we age, depression transforms into heat more readily; heat and fire tend to evaporate and consume blood and yin, and aggravate the natural predisposition to yin vacuity that is part of the process of aging.

Qi stagnation

Qi stagnation affecting the heart and lung

Disease causes, disease mechanisms: When sadness and grief remain for a long time they deplete the qi and lead to qi stagnation in the chest, which is ruled by both the heart and the lungs. Worry knots the qi and can also give rise to this pattern.

Main symptoms: A feeling of oppression and tightness in the chest, palpitations, sighing, slight breathlessness, a feeling of a lump in the throat with difficulty swallowing, pale complexion.

Symptoms associated with depression: Sadness, a tendency to weep, accompanied by anxiety, easily affected negatively by the problems of other people.

Pulse: Weak, with no wave, specially in the cun position both sides. It may also be slightly wiry, although at the same time it is vacuous and weak.

Tongue: It can be slightly red in the chest area (sides of its central section).

Treatment principles: Rectify and move the qi, stimulate the descending of heart and lung qi, and calm the spirit.

Main acupuncture points: Lu 7, Ht 7, P 6, Ren 17, Ren 15.

Additional points: St 40, LI 4, SI 5, GB 18.

Special considerations: This pattern is characterized by underlying lung qi vacuity, and possibly by heart blood vacuity in combination with liver depression. The qi stagnates primarily in the chest area, affecting the lung's function of *governing qi* (breathing and production of true qi) and to some extent the heart's function of *governing blood* (movement of blood), which are complementary to each other. There may be slight dampness or phlegm accumulation due to both lung and spleen qi vacuity. The difference between this pattern and depressive heat affecting the heart and/or lungs is that, in this case, the vacuity is more prominent and there is very slight or no depressive heat.

Qi stagnation

Blood stasis and stagnation

Disease causes, disease mechanisms: Enduring or severe liver depression may lead to an inability of the qi to move the blood; the blood becomes static because the qi is stagnant, so there is a combination of signs and symptoms of liver depression qi stagnation and symptoms of blood stasis.

Main symptoms: Abdominal distension, stabbing, fixed pain, formation of masses or swellings, dark purple, clotted bleeding (specially vaginal); dark complexion, rough, dry, and lusterless skin, with red speckles or purple macules, spider veins, prominent green-blue veins in the abdomen; in addition to signs and symptoms of qi stagnation.

Symptoms associated with depression: Vexation, agitation, thoughts of suicide, severe insomnia; chronic, recalcitrant, or severe depression.

Pulse: Fine, choppy.

Tongue: Dark, purple, with stasis speckles. Purple, distended veins under the tongue.

Treatment principles: Quicken the blood and transform stasis.

Main acupuncture points: UB 17, SP 10, SP 6, SP 8, Per 3.

Additional acupuncture points: Points used to course the liver and rectify the qi.

Special considerations: Blood stasis may result from long-standing liver depression not moving the blood, but it can also result from traumatic injury, from blood vacuity not able to nourish the vessels and keep them open, from qi vacuity not able to push the blood, or from cold congealing the blood. Because static blood hinders the creation of new or fresh blood, blood stasis may precipitate blood vacuity, and blood vacuity may precipitate blood stasis. If blood stasis is referred to the liver specifically, this means that the stasis is particularly manifest along the path traversed by the liver channel: the pelvic region, abdomen, chest, throat, and head. In depression, blood stasis either results from enduring liver depression qi stagnation or is a further complication of an underlying pattern. Blood stasis may complicate many cases of depression, especially in women who may often experience blood stasis as a factor in either the uterus, the breasts, or both.

Shen disturbance: vacuity

Heart blood and heart qi vacuity share several features in common. Before listing the features unique to each, the common features will be discussed.

General symptoms for shen disturbance caused by either heart blood or heart qi vacuity: Insomnia, heart palpitations, mild anxiety, poor memory, mild dizziness, easily startled.

General treatment principle for heart blood or heart qi vacuity patterns: Nourish the heart and calm the spirit (boost the qi and supplement the blood).

Main acupuncture points for heart blood and heart qi vacuity patterns: UB 15, UB 44, Ren 14, Ren 15, Ht 7, P 6.

Heart blood vacuity

Disease causes, disease mechanisms: As a result of constitutional insufficiency, enduring disease, aging, blood loss, or prolonged sadness and grief, there may be insufficient blood to nourish the heart.

Main symptoms: Fright palpitations, restlessness, suspiciousness, insomnia with an inability to fall asleep, excessive dreams, mild anxiety, mild dizziness, propensity to be startled, dull pale complexion, poor memory, lassitude of the spirit.

Symptoms associated with depression: Depression with fatigue, confusion, lack of concentration.

Pulse: Fine, possibly choppy.

Tongue: Pale and thin, with a thin white coat.

Treatment principles: Nourish the heart and calm the spirit, supplement the blood.

Main acupuncture points: In addition to general points above, Ren 4, St 36, Sp 6, Sp 4.

Additional acupuncture points: UB 17, Sp 10, P 7.

Special considerations: Because the spleen is the source of engenderment and transformation of both qi and blood, heart blood vacuity is commonly encountered in clinical practice in conjunction with spleen qi vacuity. This pattern is known as *heart–spleen dual vacuity* (refer to the section below on Spleen qi vacuity).

Shen disturbance: vacuity

Heart qi vacuity

Disease causes, disease mechanisms: Constitutional insufficiency, over taxation, too much thinking and worrying, sadness, grief and regret, enduring diseases, aging, blood loss.

Main symptoms: Shortness of breath and heart palpitations aggravated by exertion, insomnia, mild anxiety, poor memory, mild dizziness.

Symptoms associated with depression: Lack of motivation, fatigue and exhaustion, poor sleep.

Pulse: Fine, weak, regularly interrupted pulse.

Tongue: Pale with a thin white coating.

Treatment principles: Supplement the heart, nourish the blood, and calm the spirit.

Main acupuncture points: In addition to the main points above, Ren 4, St 36, Sp 6, Sp 4.

Additional acupuncture points: UB 20, UB 21, Du 20.

Special considerations: Heart qi vacuity is rarely seen by itself in actual clinical practice. Two subpatterns of heart qi vacuity in the Chinese Medicine literature are *heart qi not securing* (the spirit), characterized by confusion, impaired memory, easy fright, spontaneous perspiration on movement. The second subpattern is *heart qi inability to lie down*, when the heart qi is insufficient, the spirit will not be quiet, and it is difficult to lie down at night to sleep; the person is easily aroused from sleep, there are heart palpitations, a lack of strength, lassitude of spirit, aversion to cold, and a slow, forceless pulse.

Heart yin vacuity

Disease causes, disease mechanisms: Fear and worry combined with overwork for many years, aging, and congenital insufficiency may all lead to yin vacuity. In addition, enduring depressive heat may consume and evaporate blood and yin.

Main symptoms: Heart palpitations, insomnia (inability to stay asleep or waking up frequently), propensity to be startled, poor memory and concentration, anxiety, malar flush, night sweating, heat in the five centers, vexation and agitation, fidgetiness, uneasiness, restlessness, and a worsening of symptoms in the evening.

Symptoms associated with depression: Dispirited, depressed, and tired, yet anxious and restless at the same time; lack of willpower and drive.

Pulse: Rapid and thin, or floating and vacuous.

Tongue: Red tongue, redder tip, without coating.

Treatment principles: Enrich yin, settle the heart, and calm the spirit.

Main acupuncture points: UB 15, UB 44, Ren 14, Ren 15, Ht 7, P 6.

Additional acupuncture points: P 7, Kd 6, Kd 3, Kd 10, Sp 6.

Shen disturbance: vacuity

Heart fire flaming upward (heart yin vacuity with vacuity heat)

Disease causes, disease mechanisms: If depressive heat counterflows and accumulates in the heart, it may eventually consume and damage yin and blood, in which case yin will be unable to control heart yang which then becomes effulgent and hyperactive.

Main symptoms: Heart vexation, chaotic spirit, insomnia, excessive dreams, fright palpitations, racing heart, dryness of the mouth and throat, and flushing. In general, heart yin vacuity symptoms are more pronounced, anxiety and restlessness will be extreme, and the sleep will be more severely disturbed.

Symptoms associated with depression: Mentally, the person may become aggressive and very impatient.

Pulse: Floating or surging, in addition to being rapid and thready.

Tongue: Red, mirror with more pronounced redness of the tip.

Treatment principles: Enrich yin, clear heat, and drain fire; settle the heart and calm the spirit.

Main acupuncture points: Same as for yin vacuity above; in addition use Ht 6.

Special considerations: Heart fire flaming upward can be either a vacuity or repletion pattern, characterized by upper body signs (reddening of the tip of the tongue, vexation, cracking of the tongue, and erosion of the oral and glossal mucosa, rapid pulse). Here we are referring to heart fire due to heart yin vacuity, which is in turn due to kidney yin vacuity (*heart–kidney not communicating*); it is therefore necessary to supplement the kidney in order to enrich yin. As a repletion pattern, heart fire flaming upward is due to hyperactive heart fire, which in turn is due to liver fire (see below under Yang repletion patterns); in that case there is headache, red eyes, agitation, and irascibility in addition to the symptoms above. Heart fire may also spread to the small intestine, where it manifests as painful, dribbling, reddish urination.

Shen disturbance: repletion

Qi stagnation affecting the heart and lung

This is a repletion pattern that stems from a progression of liver qi stagnation, and is therefore discussed under Qi stagnation above.

Depressive heat affecting the heart or lung

This is also a repletion pattern that develops from qi stagnation transforming into heat; the disease causes, disease mechanisms, treatment principles, and points are discussed above under Liver depression transforms heat. Depressive liver heat due to emotional stress and frustration may travel upwards and accumulate in the heart and lungs. If it accumulates in the heart, it causes vexation, agitation, anxiety, insomnia, and restlessness. If it accumulates in the lungs, it causes weepiness and sadness.

Exuberant heart fire

Disease causes, disease mechanisms: Fire in the heart develops from below. It is either due to enduring emotional stress and frustration, which cause the ministerial fire to stir up and counterflow, or it is due to overeating sweet, greasy, spicy food and drinking alcohol, which cause spleen damage that leads to yin fire counterflow (see section on Yin fire in Ch. 4).

Main symptoms: Heart vexation, agitation, insomnia with excessive and disturbing dreams, racing heart, restlessness that is projected outward or is accompanied by compulsive behavior; ulcers in the mouth and on the tongue; frequent, urgent, yellow urination, dry stools, red face, red, painful, swollen, skin sores.

Symptoms associated with depression: Recurrent suicidal ideation, possibly with suicidal attempts; aggression, violent outbursts; if severe, manic agitation and delirious speech.

Pulse: Rapid, wiry, and possibly slippery or surging pulse.

Tongue: Red with a yellow coat.

Treatment principles: Clear the heart, drain fire and lead it downward, and settle the spirit.

Main acupuncture points: Ht 8, Ht 5, P 7, Ren 15, GB 15, Sp 6.

Additional acupuncture points: Du 14, LI 4, LI 11, P 8, Ht 3.

Phlegm confounding the heart (orifices)

As detailed on page 102.

Phlegm (heat) fire harassing the heart.

As detailed on page 104.

Qi/yang vacuity

Qi and yang vacuity tends to occur as a continuum, because yang is generated by the movement of qi. Yang vacuity usually implies that, in addition to signs and symptoms of qi vacuity, there is also the presence of cold.

Spleen qi (and lung qi) vacuity

Disease causes, disease mechanisms: Overwork and prolonged stress; poor diet, overeating raw and chilled foods, or undereating; overthinking and too much worry over a long period of time; chronic illness, lack of exercise.

Main symptoms: Fatigue, weakness, lethargy, loose stools, poor appetite, pale face, faint voice.

If lung qi vacuity is also present: Shortness of breath, spontaneous sweating, cough, all aggravated upon exertion.

Symptoms associated with depression: Depression with fatigue, slow thinking and speaking, slow movements, poor memory and concentration, decreased motivation, diminished interest or pleasure, excessive desire to sleep, apathy, excessive guilt, obsessive thinking or phobias, lassitude of spirit.

Pulse: Relaxed, or soggy annd weak.

Tongue: Pale, swollen, with thin white coating.

Treatment principles: Boost the qi, fortify the spleen (and the lungs).

Main acupuncture points: UB 20, UB 21, UB 49, Ren 4, Ren 6, Ren 12, St 36, Sp 3.

For lung qi vacuity: Add Lu 1, Lu 9, Lu 7, UB 13, UB 42.

Special considerations: Too much work, or even too much exercise, may consume the qi and blood, whereas too little exercise causes the qi to become stagnant. A diet of too many raw, cold, chilled foods may exhaust the digestive fire of the spleen; too many sweets, dairy products, and fried foods may also damage the spleen. As explained above, liver depression may also give rise to or exacerbate spleen vacuity. The spleen is usually the first viscus to become diseased after the liver has become depressed. If the spleen becomes vacuous and weak, it will not engender and transform the qi and blood properly, leading to vacuity of both heart blood and spleen qi (*heart–spleen dual vacuity*). If heart blood is too vacuous to nourish and quiet the spirit, the spirit may become hyperactive and restless, or it may be unable to engage the world and respond to the environment.

Qi/yang vacuity

Spleen yang vacuity

Disease causes, disease mechanisms: Enduring spleen qi vacuity or severe damage due to enduring disease; aging, or overeating raw, chilled foods.

Main symptoms: In addition to spleen qi vacuity symptoms above; edema, cold body with chilled extremities, abdominal distension and fatigue after eating, dull abdominal pain that likes warmth and pressure.

Symptoms associated with depression: More pronounced symptoms than in spleen qi vacuity.

Pulse: Sunken, forceless, or even slow.

Tongue: Swollen and pale, with teeth marks on the borders; a thin, white, slightly slimy coat.

Treatment principles: Supplement the qi and warm the spleen.

Main acupuncture points: Same as for spleen qi vacuity above. Moxa is applicable.

Kidney qi vacuity

Disease causes, disease mechanisms: Constitutional insufficiency, aging, or chronic disease; enduring spleen qi vacuity.

Main symptoms: Low back and knee soreness and weakness, premature graying or loss of hair, impotence or frigidity, uterine prolapse with weakness in the low back, frequent urination, night urination, tinnitus, dizziness, diminished auditory acuity.

Symptoms associated with depression: Mental and physical exhaustion, no willpower or initiative; hopelessness about getting better or starting or changing anything. Everything is too much effort.

Treatment principles: Nourish the kidney and supplement the qi.

Pulse: Deep and weak.

Tongue: Pale red tongue.

Main acupuncture points: UB 23, UB 52, Du 4, Ren 6, Kd 3, Kd 7.

Qi/yang vacuity

Kidney yang vacuity

Disease causes, disease mechanisms: Constitutional insufficiency, aging, or chronic disease; overwork, excessive sexual activity, or drug use.

Main symptoms: In addition to the symptoms for kidney qi vacuity above: a cold feeling in the lower part of the body, lower abdominal tension, inhibited or excessive urination, early morning diarrhea.

Symptoms associated with depression: In addition to the symptoms for kidney qi vacuity above, the person will be extremely exhausted and will lack spirits.

Treatment principles: Nourish the kidney and warm yang.

Pulse: Deep and fine in the first (chi/foot) position.

Tongue: Pale, fat, with a thin, moist coating.

Main acupuncture points: UB 23, UB 52, Du 4, Ren 6, Kd 3, Kd 7. Moxa is applicable.

Special considerations: Kidney vacuity is rarely seen alone in clinical practice; rather, it commonly combines with spleen qi vacuity to create the pattern *spleen–kidney dual vacuity*. Yang causes transformation and change; it activates and moves, and grants us the capacity to react and respond. Constitutional insufficiency, enduring disease, aging, and overwork can all lead to yang becoming vacuous. Kidney is the root of both yin and yang, providing the foundation of our life and the source of both yin and yang for all the other organs. Yang vacuity can therefore lead to vacuity of the yang of the spleen; conversely, long-standing spleen qi vacuity will lead to a depletion of kidney yang. Yang is like the fire under a kettle, if the fire is insufficient, the water in the kettle will tend to stagnate, creating a state of sogginess, congestion, inactivity, and a feeling of being frozen. Depression characterized by spleen–kidney dual vacuity will manifest as exhaustion, lack of will power and initiative, as well as hopelessness. Prolonged fear, shock, and guilt may all injure the kidney and cause this condition; but yang vacuity due to other causes can also result in fear and guilt.

Yin repletion: dampness and phlegm

Spleen vacuity, dampness accumulating

Disease causes, disease mechanisms: Due to constitutional insufficiency, chronic disease, faulty diet, overwork and too much stress, too much thinking and worry, the spleen qi may be insufficient to transport and transform liquids. It is also possible for external dampness to invade the body, causing damage to the spleen.

Main symptoms: Edema, dizziness, headache, fatigue, chest and epigastric fullness, and oppression, nausea, vomiting, diarrhea with white mucus; frequent but scanty urination; a slimy, sweet taste in the mouth.

Symptoms associated with depression: In addition to spleen qi vacuity symptoms above, mental confusion will be more severe and obsessive thinking will be more pronounced.

Pulse: A soggy, fine, and wiry pulse or a slippery, relaxed pulse.

Tongue: A swollen, pale tongue, with teeth marks on its edges and a thin, slimy, white coat.

Treatment principles: Fortify the spleen and transform dampness.

Main acupuncture points: In addition to points used to fortify the spleen above, add Sp 5, Sp 9, Ren 9.

Yin repletion: dampness and phlegm

Phlegm confounding the (orifices of the) heart

Disease causes, disease mechanisms: This pattern in mostly due to spleen vacuity and dampness engendering phlegm plus liver depression qi stagnation resulting in upward counterflow; the counterflow drafts the phlegm upwards causing mental confusion and disorientation. When such phlegm causes blockage of the flow of qi and blood to the heart, the spirit becomes much more upset. The spleen vacuity is due to a faulty diet, excessive worrying, overwork, and overthinking; the liver depression is due to anger and frustration. In addition, there may or may not be heart blood vacuity, further complicating the inability of the heart to house the spirit.

Main symptoms: Dizziness, excessive white phlegm, a feeling of oppression in the chest; no desire to eat, the sound of phlegm in the throat.

Symptoms associated with depression: Mental confusion, poor memory, withdrawal. If severe, loss of insight and total mental confusion, obsessive thinking and rumination.

Pulse: Slippery and wiry, possibly bound.

Tongue: A thick, white, slimy tongue coating.

Treatment principles: Eliminate phlegm and open the orifices of the heart.

Main acupuncture points: St 40, P 5, P 6, P 7, LI 7, LI 4, St 25, Du 20, St 8.

Additional acupuncture points: Add points that fortify the spleen, boost the qi, transform dampness, and rectify the qi.

Special considerations: This pattern occurs in several different diseases such as withdrawal disease and epilepsy. Traditionally, when this pattern refers to depression, it is characterized by severe mental confusion and disorientation, gradual appearance of abnormal behavior and dementia; this picture is more likely to be seen in patients presenting with depression with psychotic features. It is quite common, however, to encounter a milder form of this pattern in major depressive episodes. The treatment principles and treatment strategies outlined above are extremely helpful in treating major depressive episodes characterized by the presence of dampness and phlegm affecting the spirit (*shen*).

Yin repletion: dampness and phlegm

Heart vacuity, gall bladder timidity

Disease causes, disease mechanisms: Spleen vacuity causes, simultaneously, dampness and phlegm on the one hand, and blood vacuity on the other. Because the spleen qi is weak, the blood is not produced sufficiently to nourish the heart spirit, which becomes restless; the heart and lung qi are also vacuous as a result of the spleen qi being weak. At the same time, there is liver depression qi stagnation and possibly counterflow.

Symptoms associated with depression: Difficulty making decisions, lack of courage and sense of direction in life, easily startled, susceptibility to fright and fear.

Pulse: Vacuous and weak, it may be slippery in the second (guan/bar) position.

Tongue: Swollen and pale, moist coating.

Treatment principles: Warm the gall bladder, nourish the heart, and quiet the spirit.

Principal acupuncture points: GB 40, Ht 7.

Phlegm dampness obstruction and stagnation

Disease causes, disease mechanisms: The causes for this pattern are the same as those for phlegm obstructing the spirit. If in addition following the path of the liver channel, the qi becomes bound in the chest, it affects the heart and lung and causes a feeling of oppression in the chest; if the qi accumulates and counterflows, it may cause a feeling of something being stuck in the throat. In this case, phlegm and qi 'join and obstruct'.

Main symptoms: A feeling of oppression in the chest or the feeling of something stuck in the throat that can be neither spat out nor swallowed down; the person may simply experience a feeling of constant postnasal drip. Excessive phlegm that is white in color and easily expectorated, nausea, possibly vomiting, fatigue, excessive desire to sleep, possibly vertigo and palpitations.

Symptoms associated with depression: Mental confusion, tendency to ruminate and obsessive thinking, irritability and frustration.

Pulse: Wiry and slippery.

Tongue: White, slimy tongue coat.

Treatment principles: Transform phlegm, disinhibit the qi, and resolve depression.

Main acupuncture points: St 40, P 5, P 6, P 7, LI 17, LI 4.

Additional acupuncture points: Ren 17, Sp 21, St 12, GB 17, GB 18.

Yin repletion: dampness and phlegm

Phlegm fire harassing the heart

Disease causes, disease mechanisms: Basically the same as for phlegm obstructing the spirit (above), except for the addition of heat or fire arising from liver depression, qi stagnation.

Main symptoms: Emotional tension, heart vexation, agitation, red face and eyes, incessant talking, insomnia, bitter taste in the mouth, excessive or profuse yellow phlegm, chest oppression, constipation, aversion to food, burping, belching, acid regurgitation, possible nausea, vertigo, dizziness.

Symptoms associated with depression: Phlegm fire both mists and agitates the spirit. The phlegm aspect causes mental confusion, profound apathy and fatigue, poor memory; the fire aspect causes agitation, insomnia, anxiety, and in severe cases manic behavior.

Pulse: Wiry, large, rapid, slippery, possibly urgent.

Tongue: Crimson red with a thick slimy, yellow coat.

Treatment principles: Transform phlegm, clear heat, harmonize the stomach, and quiet the spirit.

Main acupuncture points: St 40, GB 15, LI, Lv 2, Ht 5, Ht 8, GB 18.

Special considerations: This mechanism is a further progression of the two mechanisms above. In this case, however, depression has endured long enough or is severe enough for liver depression to turn into depressive heat or fire. Thus there is phlegm blocking the orifices of the heart at the same time as there is fire disturbing the heart spirit. In this case, the person may alternate between periods of depression and confusion due to phlegm, and periods of abnormal elation or agitation, due to fire. This pattern, which when severe may correspond to manic depression, is very helpful in understanding the disease mechanisms that precipitate depression. It is actually extremely common to find depressive heat concomitant with dampness and phlegm accumulation. The degree of liver depression, heat or fire, and dampness or phlegm varies widely; generally, people presenting with this pattern either alternate or experience simultaneously symptoms of dampness and phlegm, such as profound apathy and lethargy, and symptoms of heat and fire, such as anxiety and agitation. Phlegm dampness obstruction and stagnation, phlegm obstructing the orifices of the heart, and phlegm fire harassing the heart lie along a continuum of a series of patterns; these patterns derive from dampness accumulation due to spleen vacuity, in combination with liver depression qi stagnation. Manic depression is a severe manifestation of this pattern, but unipolar depression accompanied by anxiety, agitation, and aggression may also be a result of this mechanism.

Additional comment on the dampness and phlegm patterns

The five depression patterns above are aggravated by faulty diet and emotional stress. Any food or drink that either damages the spleen or gives rise to more phlegm and dampness will make this disease mechanism worse. Similarly, any emotional stress or frustration making the person's liver more depressed and the qi more stagnant will exacerbate this disease mechanism.

Blood/yin vacuity

Yin and blood vacuity are considered a continuum because blood is part of yin, with the exception that blood vacuity patterns do not in themselves give rise to heat. Therefore, one important differentiation between these two patterns is the presence or absence of heat. Yin vacuity and its effects on depression depend on whether yin vacuity has given rise to vacuity heat. If there is yin vacuity only, without vacuity heat, the spirit becomes weakened and the person feels depressed, tired, and dispirited; there is mental confusion and the memory and concentration are poor. When, in addition, there is vacuity heat as a result of yin vacuity, the spirit is not only weakened but is also unsettled; the person additionally experiences anxiety and mental restlessness.

Heart blood vacuity

As detailed on page 94.

Liver blood vacuity

Disease causes, disease mechanisms: Congenital insufficiency, chronic disease, aging, excessive blood loss, prolonged anger.

Main symptoms: Mild dizziness, numbness of the limbs, early insomnia (inability to fall asleep), blurred vision, floaters in the eyes, scanty menstruation or amenorrhea, brittle nails, muscle spasms or cramps, dull pale complexion.

Symptoms associated with depression: Depression with fatigue, lack of sense of direction, in life and 'vision', confusion about own aims, fear of making decisions.

Pulse: Thin, may be choppy.

Tongue: Pale and thin, with thin white coating.

Treatment principles: Nourish the liver and supplement the blood.

Main acupuncture points: UB 17, UB 18, UB 20, UB 47, Lv 8.

Liver yin vacuity

Disease causes, disease mechanisms: Congenital insufficiency, overwork, excessive blood loss, aging, excessive sexual activity or anger, frustration and resentment over a long period of time can give rise to this pattern.

Main symptoms: Poor memory, dizziness; dry eyes, skin, and hair; blurred vision or night blindness, insomnia with restless, interrupted sleep, heat in the five centers, tidal fever, flushed cheeks in the afternoon, tremors or contractions of the sinews and muscles, numbness of the limbs, fragile nails, lateral costal pain; early, scanty, or painful menstruation.

Symptoms associated with depression: Deep depression with a lack of purpose in life, confusion about objectives and aims, restlessness. A sensation of floating before falling asleep.

Pulse: Floating and empty, or fast and wiry.

Tongue: Red tongue with no coat, or pale with red sides and tip.

Treatment principles: Nourish the liver, enrich yin, settle the hun, and quiet the spirit.

Main acupuncture points: UB 18, UB 47, Lv 8, Sp 6, Kd 3, Ren 4.

Additional points: Du 24, GB 13.

Blood/yin vacuity

Kidney yin vacuity

Disease causes, disease mechanisms: Constitutional insufficiency, age, chronic disease, overwork and prolonged emotional stress, excessive sexual activity, sequela of a febrile disease, excessive blood loss. Prolonged fear or guilt and sudden shock.

Main symptoms: Low back soreness and weakness, loss of hair, tinnitus or deafness, dizziness, low-grade afternoon fever, malar flushing, early menstruation, uterine bleeding, amenorrhea. Insomnia with difficulty staying asleep.

Symptoms associated with depression: Depression with exhaustion, lack of willpower, feeling aimless; rigid mental attitude, restlessness, fidgety, despair.

Pulse: Deep, fine, and rapid.

Tongue: Red tongue, with a thin, yellow, scanty, dry or absent coating.

Treatment principles: Supplement the kidney and enrich yin.

Main acupuncture points: UB 23, UB 52, Kd 3, Kd 6, Kd 10, Sp 6, Ren 4.

Additional points: Kd 9, Kd 22, Kd 27.

Lung yin vacuity

Disease causes, disease mechanisms: Same as for kidney yin vacuity. Kidney yin vacuity and lung yin vacuity may give raise to each other or appear simultaneously. Lung yin vacuity may also be precipitated by sadness and grief.

Main symptoms: Same as for kidney yin vacuity, with the addition of dry cough with scanty phlegm, chronic low-grade sore throat, dry skin, with skin rashes.

Symptoms associated with depression: In addition to symptoms of kidney yin vacuity above, melancholy, sadness, and a tendency to hang on to the past nostalgically.

Pulse: Fine and floating.

Tongue: Red tongue with scanty coating.

Treatment principles: Supplement the lung (and kidney), enrich yin.

Main acupuncture points: In addition to points for kidney yin vacuity, add UB 13, UB 42, Lu 9, Lu 5, Lu 7 (with Kd 6).

Yang repletion and vacuity heat

Liver depression transforms heat

As seen above, this pattern develops from liver depression qi stagnation, and is therefore described in full under that section.

Hyperactivity of liver yang

Disease causes, disease mechanisms: Kidney yin vacuity due to constitutional insufficiency, aging, long-term or severe disease, too much work, excessive sexual activity or sexual desire may give rise to hyperactivity of liver yang or ascendant fire. Anything that speeds up the body or pushes the body to prolonged excessive activity may lead to yin vacuity and yang hyperactivity, such as caffeinated drinks, recreational drugs, and too much exercise. Any of these can waste yin and stir yang hyperactively. Enduring stress may cause prolonged liver depression to transform into heat; this heat may eventually consume blood and body fluids, and damage yin. Depleted yin becomes unable to control yang, and yang counterflows upward, with symptoms of heat and repletion above and of cold and vacuity below.

Main symptoms: Headache, dizziness, vertigo, tinnitus, low back ache.

Symptoms associated with depression: Pronounced irritability, palpitations, insomnia, and anxiety.

Pulse: Wiry and rapid.

Tongue: Red.

Treatment principles: Pacify the liver and subdue rebellious yang; clear heat, quicken the blood, supplement and boost the liver and kidney.

Main acupuncture points: GB 20, Lv 2, Lv 3, LI 11, Yintang.

Additional acupuncture points: Sp 6, TH 5, GB 43, Kd 3.

Special considerations: In depression, this pattern rarely occurs on its own. Generally, one encounters anxiety, agitation, and severe insomnia as manifestations of yin vacuity, fire effulgence, concomitant with spleen qi, kidney yang vacuity (spleen–kidney dual vacuity); the latter gives rise to dampness and phlegm, which precipitates some of the apathy, lethargy, and anhedonia characteristic of depression.

Yang repletion and vacuity heat

Liver fire flaming upward

Disease causes: Emotional stress, frustration, and anger may cause enduring liver depression, which transforms into heat. If this heat becomes exacerbated it can turn into fire and flare upward, affecting the liver and its associated channels and network vessels. Overeating hot, greasy, and fatty foods, and alcohol, can give rise to dampness, which precipitates downward to the liver channel and causes damp heat in the lower burner; the heat may also draft the dampness upwards in the form of phlegm, obstructing the heart and agitating the spirit.

Main symptoms: Red face and eyes, bitter taste in the mouth, dry mouth, headache, dizziness, tinnitus and deafness, scorching pain on the ribs.

Symptoms associated with depression: Very angry, prone to outbursts of anger, impatience, restlessness, irritability; insomnia with violent dreams, vexation, and agitation. If the anger is harbored inside for many years, this may lead to depression, which looks like sadness and grief, but is in fact anger.

Pulse: Rapid and forceful, or rapid, slippery, and wiry.

Tongue: Red with a slimy yellow coat.

Treatment principles: Clear the liver and drain fire, quiet the spirit, and settle the hun.

Main acupuncture points: Lv 2, Lv 3, UB 18, Sp 6, Du 18, Du 24, GB 13, GB 15.

Additional acupuncture points: Ht 5, Ht 8.

Yang repletion and vacuity heat

Yin vacuity, fire effulgence (vacuity heat)

Disease causes, disease mechanisms: If, as a result of constitutional insufficiency, aging, enduring disease, overtaxation or excessive sexual activity, yin becomes insufficient, it may be unable to control yang, and therefore fire counterflows upward. In this case, the fire stems from yin vacuity and is severe.

Main symptoms: Night sweats, tidal fever, heat in the five centers, increased sexual libido, heart palpitations, malar flush, dizziness, tinnitus, frequent urination, with scant, yellow urine; red lips, dry throat; vertigo and dizziness; possibly seminal emission in men and irregular periods in women.

Symptoms associated with depression: Fearfulness, anxiety, restlessness, insomnia, heart vexation, easy anger, symptoms worst in the evening, fidgetiness, hypersensitivity.

Pulse: Fine, rapid, and possibly floating, specially in the first (inch/cun) position.

Tongue: A red tongue with scanty yellow coating.

Treatment principles: Enrich yin, clear heat or drain fire, settle the heart, and calm the spirit.

Main acupuncture points: UB 23, Kd 3, Kd 10, Sp 6.

Additional acupuncture points: Ht 6, SI 3.

Special considerations: The patterns hyperactivity of liver yang, yin vacuity–fire effulgence, vacuity heat or fire, and yin vacuity–heat effusion (not mentioned here) are all variations of a basic disease mechanism in which there is insufficiency of yin, and repletion of heat or fire due to or exacerbated by this insufficiency. Yin vacuity originates from the kidney and may affect the other viscera and bowels; the heat or fire may arise from the liver, the heart, or the stomach and consume yin; alternatively, it may arise from the yin insufficiency itself, and flare upwards or exacerbate an underlying accumulation of heat.

Yang repletion and vacuity heat

Spleen vacuity giving rise to fire (yin fire)

Disease causes, disease mechanisms: Overthinking and worry, overworking, faulty diet and poor eating habits damage the spleen; if the spleen fails to control transportation and transformation it gives rise to dampness which percolates downward and damages the liver and kidneys. Dampness accumulation often transforms into damp heat. Dampness damages the kidney yang and the heat of damp heat tends to float upward; yang loses its root in its lower source (kidneys) and also tends to surge upwards.

Main symptoms: Fatigue, lassitude of the spirit, weak extremities, lower back ache, low sexual desire, incontinence of urine, cold extremities, possibly unusual vaginal discharge or genital itching, turbid urination.

Symptoms associated with depression: Sorrow, inexplicable weeping and crying, agitation, anxiety, and insomnia.

Pulse: Large, slippery, floating, and rootless, especially in the first (cun/inch) position.

Tongue: Swollen, tooth-marked, dark hue, thicker yellow coat in the back, red tip.

Treatment principles: Supplement the spleen, transform dampness, rectify the qi, and clear heat.

Main acupuncture points: Ren 4, Ren 6, Ren 15, UB 20, UB 23, Sp 9, Sp 6, Ht 5.

Additional acupuncture points: Depend on the specific presenting signs and symptoms.

Special considerations: This pattern is a result of the complex mechanisms known as *yin fire*. Yin fire is different from vacuity heat (effulgent fire due to yin vacuity). Yin fire is a condition where yin cold and dampness are generated by a damaged spleen. Due to overthinking and worry, overworking, or faulty diet and eating habits, the spleen fails to control transportation and transformation. The turbid portion of foods and liquids is not separated from the clear, and this becomes damp turbidity. This damp turbidity, which is yin, percolates downward, damaging the liver and kidneys. Because the host qi of the body is yang, yang turbidity often transforms into damp heat; dampness damages kidney yang, and both the heat of damp heat and the yang of the kidney tend to float and surge upwards. Usually there are symptoms of cold (and possibly also damp heat) in the lower body, as well as symptoms of heat in the upper part of the body, with other symptoms manifesting as weakness of the spleen. In the case of depression, this fire can either disturb the lungs giving rise to sorrow, inexplicable weeping, and crying, or it can disturb the heart giving rise to agitation, inappropriate laughter, and insomnia. This heat can also affect the stomach, precipitating insomnia and in severe cases manic symptoms.

The 12 Main Basic Patterns and Pattern Combinations

The 12 main basic patterns and pattern combinations are shown in Box 5.1.

BOX 5.1	*Basic patterns and pattern combinations*
	1. Liver depression qi stagnation
	2. Liver depression transforms heat (including depressive heat affecting the heart and lung)
	3. Liver qi stagnation affecting the heart and lung
	4. Liver stagnation and stasis
	5. Heart–spleen dual vacuity (heart blood–spleen qi vacuity)
	6. Spleen–kidney dual vacuity (spleen qi–kidney yang vacuity)
	7. Phlegm confounding the orifices of the heart
	8. Heart vacuity, gall bladder timidity
	9. Phlegm dampness obstruction and stagnation
	10. Phlegm fire harassing the heart
	11. Yin vacuity, fire effulgence
	12. Spleen vacuity giving rise to fire

STRATEGIES AND TECHNIQUES

Points, Point Combinations, and Their Use in Major Depression

Patterns of disharmony rarely, if ever, happen on their own. Clinically, a combination of two or more patterns forms a complex web of interactions and interrelations. In depression, the combination of patterns incorporates elements of the four features on which this framework is based: (1) qi stagnation, (2) shen disturbance (vacuity or repletion), (3) vacuity of qi/yang and/or repletion of dampness/phlegm, (4) vacuity of yin/blood and/or repletion of heat/fire.

To arrive at a set of treatment principles and develop a treatment strategy, the patterns of disharmony involved, as well as their interactions and interrelations, must be identified. This is where the skill of the practitioner comes into play: to weave all the pertinent information into a complete symptom picture and, with this information, develop a treatment approach.

The assessment questionnaire developed for the study (see Appendix A) outlines the main symptoms for each pattern; because it is not a linear process, some overlap and some omissions are inevitable. The qualified practitioner takes this information to create a pattern of disharmony, and then uses this pattern as a guideline to develop a treatment protocol. The rationale for arriving at a particular treatment strategy needs to be outlined clearly. This is essential so that the practitioner can evaluate treatment progress; if the treatment fails, it will help the practitioner to determine why it may not be yielding the expected results. It is also important for allowing other practitioners to follow the rationale and assess the suitability of the diagnosis and treatment.

For example, assume a client presents with depression characterized by depressed mood with both irritability and lethargy. Additionally she experiences breast distension, premenstrual exacerbation of emotional lability, edema and fatigue after eating, insomnia with an inability to fall asleep, and an increased desire to sleep during the day; her pulse is wiry but also soggy in the second position on the right, and her tongue is swollen, pale, with darker sides and a red tip.

The first step involves differentiation of signs and symptoms:

- depressed mood with both irritability and lethargy: liver depression qi stagnation, spleen qi vacuity

- breast distension, premenstrual emotional lability: liver depression qi stagnation

- edema and fatigue after eating: dampness accumulation due to spleen vacuity

- insomnia with an inability to fall asleep: heart blood vacuity

- increased desire to sleep: qi vacuity, dampness accumulation

- wiry pulse: liver depression qi stagnation

- soggy pulse in the second right position: spleen qi vacuity

- puffy pale tongue: spleen qi vacuity, blood vacuity

- darker sides of tongue: liver depression qi stagnation

- red tip of tongue: shen disturbance due to heat agitating the heart.

Second, identify the pattern(s) of disharmony. This combination of signs and symptoms points to liver depression qi stagnation, heart–spleen dual vacuity, dampness accumulation due to spleen vacuity.

Third, establish the treatment principles. Course the liver, rectify the qi, and boost the qi, strengthen the spleen, nourish the heart (and blood), and calm the spirit.

Finally, select the points:

- to course the liver, rectify the qi: LV 3 and LI 4

- to boost the qi and strengthen the spleen: Ren 4, St 36, UB 20, SP 6

- to nourish the heart and calm the spirit: UB 15, Ht 7, P 6.

A first treatment, then, might include the following points: Lv 3 bilateral, LI 4 on the right, P 6 on the left, HT 7 on the left, Ren 4, ST 36 bilateral, Sp 6 bilateral.

The decision to needle the points contralaterally[1] instead of bilaterally is made on the basis of the clinical findings (signs and symptoms, tongue, pulse). The treatments and the sequence of treatments throughout the sessions are selected on the basis of severity and number of symptoms for each category (i.e. qi stagnation, shen disturbance, qi vacuity), as well as on the basis of an understanding of the disease mechanisms that precipitate specific patterns. Points are selected for their specific actions and their most effective combinations.

GUIDELINES FOR TREATMENT DESIGN

The points listed under each pattern above are given only as guidelines to address the treatment principles. To design successful treatments, one must choose from the lists of points and create effective point combinations, which address the specific pattern interactions for each client. The point functions and indications are based on *The Practice of Chinese Medicine* (Maciocia 1994).

Within the parameters of a research study, and in order to facilitate reliability and replicability, clear guidelines must be established in the selection of points. Furthermore, needling techniques must be standardized and consistent (neutral stimulation being the most easily replicable technique in a research setting). Without the additional benefit of specific needling techniques, effective point combinations are even more essential. The guidelines for point selection and needling techniques must allow the practitioner sufficient flexibility to provide an individually tailored treatment, while keeping in line with the stated framework.

In our research protocol, neutral stimulation and standard angle insertion (Xinnong 1987) were selected; needles were retained for 20 minutes, unless otherwise specified. Assessing acupuncturists (who design the treatment plans) were asked to adhere to the list of points and not to add points or combinations not included in the manual.

Because of the nature of the study design, which involved separating the assessment from the treatment, the assessing acupuncturists

[1]The term contralaterally, when used in this text, implies a point used unilaterally in relationship to another point needled on the opposite side as well as the opposite extremity, e.g. a point on the left foot needled in conjunction with a point on the right arm.

were asked to design a series of treatments to be used over time (8 weeks). These series needed to address effectively the complete set of treatment principles for treating the pattern combination and disease mechanisms appropriate for each person. For this reason, guidelines for point combinations, as well as guidelines for designing treatment progressively over time, have been outlined.

To design the most effective treatments there are four factors that must be taken into consideration in the selection and combination of points, which are described more fully in Maciocia (1994):

1. The dynamics of the flow of qi in the channels (according to their position and dynamics within the channel system)

2. The energetic action of the point (their particular action, function, nature, or quality)

3. The combination of points from different channels (to address the complex pattern combination and disease mechanisms)

4. The area of the body affected by the point.

The Dynamics of the Flow of Qi in the Channels

It is important always to balance local and distal, upper and lower, left and right. Later on, the use of specific guidelines in combining points following our protocol will be described in detail.

Local and Distal

Local points (L) include the head and trunk. Distal points (D) include the arms below the elbows, and the legs below the knees. Examples are shown in Box 5.2.

Upper and Lower

Upper points (U) include the arms, and lower points (L) include the legs; the combination of upper and lower points allows the balance of yin–yang channels, greater units (taiyin, shaoyang, jueyin), etc. Examples are given in Box 5.3.

Left and Right

This is an extremely important tool that allows us to create dynamic treatment strategies. Maciocia (1994) says that needling points contralaterally is 'like applying a force to the tangents of two opposite

BOX 5.2	Balance of local and distal points	
	To course the liver, rectify the qi:	(L) Lv 14, UB 18 (D) Lv 3–P 6
	To stimulate the descending of lung qi:	(L) Sp 21, Ren 17 (D) Lu 7, P 6
	To stimulate the descending of heart qi:	(L) Ren 15, Ren 14 (D) Ht 7, P 6
	To nourish the heart and calm the spirit:	(L) UB 15, UB 44, Ren 14, Ren 15 (D) Ht 7, P 6
	To fortify the spleen and boost the qi:	(L) UB 20, Ren, 12, Ren 6, Ren 4 (D) St 36, Sp 3, Sp 4
	To harmonize the heart, clear heat, drain fire and settle the spirit:	(L) Ren 14, Ren 15, UB 15, UB 14 (D) Ht 5, HT 8–GB 15
	To supplement the kidney:	(L) Ren 6, UB 23, UB 52 (D) KD 3, KD 7, KD 9
	To supplement the kidney and enrich yin:	(L) KD 22, KD 27, UB 23 (D) KD 3, KD 6, KD 10
	To pacify the liver, subdue rebellious yang, and clear heat:	(L) LV 14, UB 18, UB 47 (D) LV 2, LI 11, GB 20

BOX 5.3	Balance of upper and lower points	
	To course the liver, rectify the qi, resolve depression, open the chest, settle the ethereal soul (hun):	(U) P 6–Lv 3 (L) (U) LI 4–LV 3 (L) (U) P 7–LV 3 (L)
	To transform dampness, eliminate phlegm, and open the orifices of the heart:	(U) P 6–ST 40 (L)
	To supplement the kidney, (enrich yin), settle the heart, and calm the spirit:	(U) HT 7–KD 3 (L) (U) HT 6–KD 7 (L) (U) HT 7–KD 9 (L)

poles of a circle, making it spin' (p. 828). Seem (1985) describes it as setting in motion the flow of qi in the channels in an infinite (∞) pattern. Points can be combined and needled contralaterally.

- When intended to move qi and blood: Lv 3 (R)–LI 4 or P6 (L); or Sp 4 (R)–P 6 (L)

- To balance arm and leg channels of the same polarity (spleen and lung, heart and kidney, liver and pericardium, etc.): KD 3 (L)–Ht 7, Ht 5 (R); or LV 3 (R)–P 6, P 5, P 4 (L)

- To balance exteriorly–interiorly related channels (lung–large intestine, spleen–stomach, kidney–bladder): TB 6 (R)–P 6 (L); or TB 3 (L)–P 7 (R); or HT 7 (L)–SI 5 (R)

- To balance extraordinary vessels (du mo, ren mo, chung mo, yin wei mo, etc.): Sp 4 (L)–P 6 (R); or GB 41 (R)–TH 5 (L)

- To balance divergent channels (although divergent channels are not used in this protocol)

- To balance connecting channels (i.e. using connecting and source points): LI 4 (L)–Lu 7 (R); or P 6 (R)–TH 4 (L); or ST 40 (L)–SP 3 (R)

- To balance unrelated yin and yang channels, to achieve effective point combinations: St 40 (R)–P 5 (L); or GB 40 (L)–Ht 7 (R)

It is important to note that this is a sample list of how points may be combined; some of the point combinations listed above have not been used as part of our protocol. For a complete list of treatment principles and the point options used in this protocol, refer to Table 5.1B & C (Treatment principles and Points for each pattern). For a more complete list of effective point combinations, refer to the following section.

The Action of Points and Special Point Combinations Useful in the Treatment of Depression

Box 5.4 provides a list of points and special point combinations that have direct effects on the treatment of symptoms encountered in depression. Each point or combination is listed with its intended effect.

BOX 5.4		Points and point combinations useful in the treatment of depression
	UB 42	PO HU	Strengthens and roots the corporeal soul (po). Frees up breathing when worry, sadness, and grief constrict the po. Calms spirit, settles the corporeal soul (po). Makes person turn inward and be comfortable with one.
	UB 44	SHENTANG	Nourishes the heart and calms spirit. Left for longer than 15 minutes, clears heart fire. Stimulates intelligence and mental clarity.
	UB 47	HUNMEN	Settles and roots the ethereal soul (hun). Strengthens the hun's capacity for planning, sense of aim in life, life's dreams and projects.

BOX 5.4		*Points and point combinations useful in the treatment of depression (contd)*	
			Like a door, facilitates the coming and going of the hun. Best combined with UB 23 and 52, to prevent it from making the hun too mobile and unsettled, and the patient shaky and insecure (especially in people who are too open, unstable, or vulnerable). Physically, it helps to treat liver qi stagnation insulting the lungs.
UB 49	YISHE		Strengthens the intellect, clears spirit, and stimulates memory and concentration. Relieves obsessive thinking, brooding, rumination.
UB 52	ZHISHI		Strengthens willpower, drive, determination, capacity to pursue one's goals with single-mindedness, spirit of initiative, steadfastness. In combination with other UB outer line points, used as a solid mental–emotional foundation for the other aspects of the psyche; in this case it is also paired up with UB 23.
		With UB 42	Strengthens willpower and drive, settles po, and releases emotions.
		With UB 44	Strengthens willpower and drive, calms the spirit, and relieves anxiety, depression, mental restlessness, and insomnia.
		With UB 47	Strengthens willpower and drive, instills a sense of direction and aim in life. Used in chronic depression to treat mental exhaustion, lack of drive, and aimlessness.
		With UB 49	Strengthens willpower and drive, and clears obsessive thoughts, worries, and confused thinking.
Du 18	QIANGJIANG		Opens the heart's orifices and calms spirit. Regulates liver blood. Severe mental restlessness, agitation, confusion, and obsessive thoughts due to blood stasis.
Du 19	HOUDING		Calms spirit and strengthens willpower. Used in severe anxiety and mental restlessness due to kidney vacuity with vacuity heat.
		With Ren 15	Calms the spirit, relieves anxiety, insomnia, and mental restlessness.
Du 20	BAIHUI		Clears spirit, lifts the mood, and stimulates memory and concentration.

BOX 5.4	*Points and point combinations useful in the treatment of depression (contd)*		
	Du 21	QIANTING	Strengthens the spirit. Treats slight anxiety, insomnia, and depression.
	Du 24	SHENTING	Stimulates intelligence, and clears the mind.
		With GB 13	Calms the mind, settles the hun. To treat anxiety, mental restlessness due to liver disharmonies.
	Ren 15	JIUWEI	Calms the spirit, settles the po. Releases emotions constraining the po in the chest and causing a feeling of oppression or tightness in the chest. Can be a very calming point, especially in conditions due to vacuity.
		With Du 19	Calms the spirit, relieves anxiety, insomnia, and mental restlessness.
	Ren 4	GUANYUAN	Strengthens the willpower and calms the spirit. Roots the spirit in the kidney, 'grounding' it. Used to treat anxiety and mental restlessness in kidney vacuity.
	GB 13	BENSHEN	Calms the spirit, settles the hun; gathers essence to the head. Relieves severe anxiety and mental restlessness due to liver disharmony. Reduces jealousy and suspicion. Improves mental clarity due to injury of the hun by sadness.
		With Du 24	As described above, enhances its calming effect.
		With Ht 7	Calms the spirit in severe anxiety due to heart disharmony.
	GB 15	TOULINQI	Calms the spirit, settles the hun. Reduces emotional fluctuations and obsessive thinking.
	GB 17	ZHENGYING	Calms and clears the spirit. Stimulates memory and concentration.
	GB 18	CHENGLING	Settles the hun and po, and stops obsessive thoughts. Physically stimulates the dispersing and descending of lung qi and opens the nose.
	GB 40	QIUXU	Strengthens the willpower and the spirit. Bolsters the capacity to make decisions.
	Ht 7	SHENMEN	Calms and nourishes the spirit. Specially indicated in heart blood and heart yin vacuity.

BOX 5.4		*Points and point combinations useful in the treatment of depression (contd)*
Ht 6	YINXI	Calms the spirit. Repletion patterns with vacuity heat.
Ht 8	SHAOFU	Calms the spirit. Reduces severe mental restlessness, anxiety, and insomnia from repletion patterns such as heart fire, phlegm fire.
Ht 9	SHAOCHONG	Same as Ht 8 above.
P 7	DAILING	Calms the spirit, especially in repletion patterns. Resolves heart phlegm. Specially indicated for emotional problems from the breaking of relationships. Has an inward movement.
P 6	NEIGUAN	Calms the spirit, lifts mood, relaxes the chest. Rectifies the qi. Specially indicated for emotional problems associated with qi stagnation. Settles the hun and calms the spirit when they are affected by anger, resentment, or frustration. Releases constrained emotions in the chest, with a feeling of oppression or tightness. Has an outward movement, moves the qi, resolves stagnation, and 'opens' the spirit.
	With Sp 4	Opens yin wei mo, nourishes blood, relaxes the chest, calms the spirit, and settles the hun.
	With Lv 3	Strengthens its qi rectification action in emotional problems from repressed anger.
	With Du 20	Lifts the mood, clears the spirit, relieves depression.
	With Du 26	Lifts the mood, clears the spirit, opens the heart orifices, and relieves depression.

Source: Maciocia (1994), with permission.

Point Combinations from Different Channels

The following section summarizes the actions of point combinations, involving points from different channels. They emphasize functions of the viscera and bowels involved in depression.

■ To harmonize heart and kidney, nourish the heart (enrich yin), and calm the spirit: Ht 7–KD 3
  – In addition, to clear vacuity heat (and stop night sweating): Ht 6–KD 7

- To enrich yin further and clear vacuity heat: Ht 5–KD 6
- In addition to relieve oppression in the chest (very calming point combination): Ht 7–KD 9
- To clear heat further from the heart (depressive, replete, or vacuity heat): Ht 5–KD 9

■ To harmonize Jueyin (Lv/Per), regulate qi, open the chest, resolve depression, release suppressed emotions, and settle the hun: Lv 3–P 6
- In addition, to calm the spirit and/or eliminate phlegm and open orifices of the heart: Lv 3–P 7
- To regulate the descending of Lu/Ht qi, clear depressive heat affecting the Ht/Lu, settle the heart, and calm the spirit: Lv 3–P 4

■ To course the liver, rectify the qi, resolve depression, calm the spirit, settle the ethereal soul, and regulate the ascendance and descendance of qi: Lv 3–LI 4 (Note: Avoid this combination during pregnancy.)

■ To regulate the middle burner, subdue counterflow qi, resolve phlegm, calm the spirit: P 6–St 40
- In addition, to open the orifices of the heart add: GB 18
- In addition, to clear heat and drain fire from the heart add: Ht 5, Ht 8
- In addition, to clear heat: P 5–St 40

■ To regulate the middle burner and subdue counterflow qi, concomitant with spleen–stomach vacuity: P 6–St 36

■ To strengthen memory and concentration due to spleen–heart dual vacuity: Ht 5–Sp 3

■ To nourish the heart, calm the spirit, and open the orifices of the heart. To assist decision-making by discriminating between choices: Ht 7–SI 5

■ To course the liver, rectify the qi, settle the ethereal soul, when distension combines physically with emotional moodiness and depression: Lv 3–GB 34[2]

■ To fortify the spleen, boost the qi, and nourish the blood: St 36–Sp 6 (Note: Needle both points bilaterally.)

■ To course the liver, rectify the qi, and resolve depression, when it causes chest oppression and sighing: P 6–TH 6

■ To course the liver, rectify the qi, open the orifices of the heart, calm the spirit, and lift the mood, when the patient presents with mental

[2](Note: Needle Lv on one side, contralaterally to another complementary point (i.e. P 6), and needle GB 34 bilaterally.)

confusion and depression due to long-standing emotional problems and suppressed emotions: P 6–TH 3

■ For the same indications as the previous combination, with a more calming effect: P 7–TH 3

■ To course the liver, rectify the qi, calm the spirit, resolve counterflow qi headaches, neck tension due to emotional problems: P 6–TH 4

■ To nourish the heart, calm the spirit, and strengthen the gall bladder's capacity to make decisions: GB 40–Ht 7.

According to the Areas of the Body Affected by the Points

When selecting distal points, it is important to consider the area affected by the point, in addition to considering the action of the points or the dynamics of the flow of qi in the channels (Maciocia 1994). The general principle is that the further the point is along the channel, the further its influence is exerted; this is true only for the points on the arms and the legs, which affect the upper extremity of the channels. For a detailed overview of the areas affected by the principal channel points, see Maciocia (1994).

SPECIAL CONSIDERATIONS WHEN TREATING DEPRESSION DURING PREGNANCY

It is traditionally stated in Chinese Medicine that acupuncture should be performed conservatively during pregnancy in order to minimize the possibility of inducing miscarriage or precipitating premature labor. If performed judiciously, knowledgeably, and with care, however, it can be extremely beneficial as a remedial treatment for a number of problems that may arise during pregnancy, including depression. Caution must be employed to avoid any points forbidden during pregnancy, unless they clearly readdress a complication of pregnancy (Flaws 1983). The application of this framework in research protocols during depression in pregnancy should avoid the following points:

With needle LI 4, Sp 1, Sp 6, GB 21, UB 60, UB 67, Ren 3, 4, 5, and 6
With moxa LI 4, Sp 2, Ren 3, 4, 5, and 6

In addition, the following points are advised against: St 36, St 45, UB 23, UB 32, Kd 4, GB 44, Lv 1 (moxa).

These points either directly or indirectly create a lot of movement in the pelvic cavity, and some affect the uterus specifically; they can potentially create an unnecessary stirring of the fetus, which could lead to miscarriage or premature labor. Many of these points are in fact used to promote labor.

GUIDELINES FOR TREATMENT DELIVERY

In our research protocol, we adhered to the following guidelines in the delivery of treatment:

1. Only use points outlined in the manual and preferably use points in combinations that include more than just one function.

2. Address two or more treatment principles simultaneously with fewer needles, by needling two sets of points contralaterally; for example, liver depression, qi stagnation affecting the heart and lung, kidney vacuity, heart yin vacuity with vacuity heart: Lv 3 (R)–P 6 (L) or LI 4 (L); or KD 3 (L)–Ht 6 (R).

3. Use a balanced combination of local and distal points. Needle local points bilaterally when appropriate. In the example above, add Sp 21 bilaterally or Ren 17 or Ren 15.

4. Always needle bilaterally points that are intended to supplement and nourish. In the example above, one could add Sp 6 bilaterally, UB 23 bilaterally, or needle KD 3 bilaterally instead.[3]

5. Add at least one point to lift the mood further, resolve depression, calm the spirit and/or open the orifices of the heart, as appropriate. In the example above, one could add Du 19.

6. If more than one treatment is being given per week, for example at the beginning when more frequent treatments are indicated, it is helpful to maintain the same strategy throughout the week and have the option to *alternate* or *choose* between two points that have a similar and complementary function. Only choose or alternate between *two points that have similar indications when in combination to the whole treatment*. For example:

   Sp 21 choose/alternate Ren 17; Ren 4 choose/alternate Ren 6 or UB 20, UB 23; and P 6 choose/alternate LI 4.

   Do not choose or alternate between two points meant to be used in combination with each other, such as LV 3–P 6.

---

[3]In pregnant women, abdominal points will be avoided as outlined in the guidelines for treatment during pregnancy. Remember that pregnant women will likely be treated lying on their side, in which case one could do a set of back shu points and a front mu point.

7. Design treatment plans to address *over time* (the entire duration of the treatment; i.e. 8 weeks,) *all* the treatment principles outlined in the pattern differentiation (based on the presenting signs and symptoms, constitution of the patient, rate of severity, previous history of depression, etc.).

8. During the first 4 weeks of treatment emphasize coursing the liver, rectifying the qi, transforming dampness and phlegm, clearing heat, calming the spirit, etc., and secondarily treat the underlying vacuity. After that, focus on fortifying the spleen, boosting the qi, nourishing the heart, supplementing the kidneys, etc., while continuing to address the other disease mechanisms.

9. In menstruating women, emphasize coursing, rectifying, transforming, and clearing in the 2 weeks preceding the menstrual cycle. Focus on boosting, supplementing, nourishing, and fortifying in the week after the period. During menstruation it is best to continue with the premenstrual strategy, except towards the end of the period.

10. Use mu points and other points on the ventral aspect of the body for the first 2 weeks and then use shu points. Use the points on the outer line of the UB channel, after having addressed the main patterns, on both the ventral and dorsal aspects of the body (around week 4, treatment 7).

11. Use a total of seven acupuncture points and three auricular points.

   a. Select the seven acupuncture points from a set of five main points that together address the appropriate combination of the four main features: (1) liver depression qi stagnation, (2) shen disturbance due to vacuity or repletion, (3) vacuity of qi–yang/blood–yin, and/or (4) repletion of dampness–phlegm or hyperactivity of yang.

   b. Select at least one of the two remaining points to regulate the du channel or directly affect mental functions (i.e. Du 24 or GB 18), and the other point to address the pattern differentiation further.

   c. Select three auricular points from the list provided, based on the *Auriculotherapy Manual* (Oleson 1992) (see Table 5.2 and Fig. 5.1), to further address damage by the emotions.

   d. The treatment course consists of 12 acupuncture treatments given over an 8-week period, biweekly for the first 4 weeks and weekly during the next 4 weeks.

FIGURE 5.1   *Auricular points commonly used in depression*

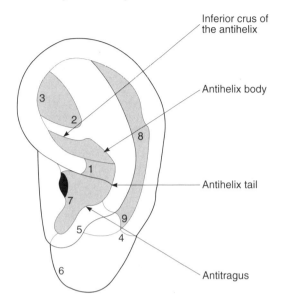

Inferior crus of the antihelix

Antihelix body

Antihelix tail

Antitragus

The location for the auricular points used in the protocol were selected from the Auriculotherapy Manual *(Oleson 1992).*

e. Although in our original study no maintenance or follow-up phase was built in, it is strongly advised to follow the acute treatment phase with maintenance treatments. Maintenance may involve two acupuncture treatments per month for 3 months, then one treatment per month for the following 3 months, with a seasonal tune-up treatment every time the season changes.

ASSESSMENT: SPECIAL CONSIDERATIONS REGARDING THE USE OF THE FOUR EVALUATIONS IN ASSESSING DEPRESSION

Framework

As mentioned in Chapter 3, the theoretical framework presented in this book focuses primarily on the use of three of the five filters – (1) eight principles, (2) viscera and bowels, (3) qi, blood, and body fluids, – with additional consideration of the five phases in the assessment interview, and a broad inclusion of channel interactions in the design of treatment protocols. The integration of all five levels is ideal; this manual represents our own particular effort towards developing a

FIGURE 6.1 Tanya's tongue

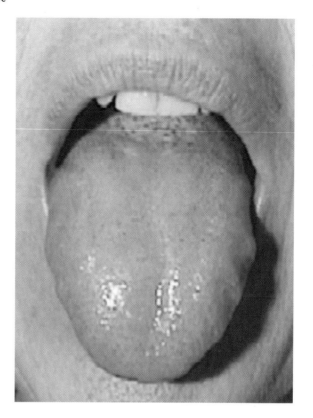

FIGURE 6.2 Karen's tongue

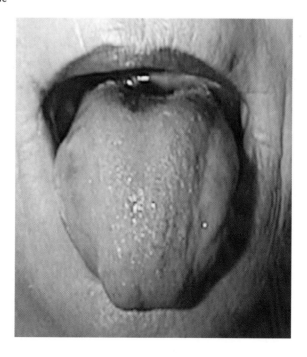

FIGURE 6.3 Francesca's tongue

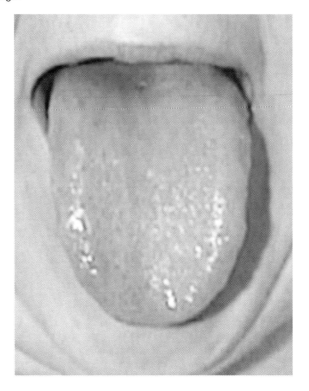

FIGURE 6.4 Tim's tongue

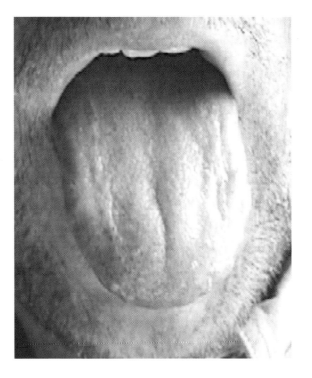

multidimensional approach to the treatment of depression based on the principles of Chinese Medicine.

In the protocol presented here, after conducting an assessment with the four evaluations, the presenting signs and symptoms are differentiated on the basis of the four features as detailed below. It is also necessary to assess the specific viscera and bowels involved.

Liver Depression Qi Stagnation

The level of liver depression qi stagnation is evaluated, as are the level of heat transformation and the degree to which the stagnation may be affecting either the heart or the lung. Points are then chosen to course the liver and rectify the qi, clear heat, calm the *shen*, and assist in descending lung qi accordingly. In menstruating women, mood and symptom changes related to the menstrual cycle are considered important factors because of the liver's effect on the movement of blood. Premenstrually, emphasis is placed on coursing the liver, rectifying the qi, and clearing heat, as appropriate (i.e. treating the repletion caused or aggravated by stagnation). Postmenstrually, emphasis is placed on supplementing vacuity. This is based on the understanding that repletion symptoms typically manifest before menstruation and vacuity symptoms manifest after menstruation. As explained in the section on the menstrual cycle, yang begins to grow during the third week of the cycle, and qi and blood are both at their maximum in the week preceding menstruation. The blood becomes relatively empty as part of the process of menstruation, being most vacuous at the conclusion of the period (Flaws 1992). Again, we determine to what extent the stagnation has transformed into heat (repletion of yang), whether it has given rise to blood stasis, or whether it has caused dampness and phlegm to accumulate. We believe that this information can potentially help to predict outcome and relapse, based on the hypothesis that the greater degree of blood stasis and phlegm accumulation, the lower the rate of remission and the higher the incidence of relapse, given acupuncture treatment alone.

Shen Disturbance

The nature and degree of shen disturbance is examined to determine whether it is due to vacuity (heart blood, heart qi, or heart yin vacuity with or without vacuity heat) or to repletion (qi stagnation, or depressive heat affecting the heart, or phlegm confounding the orifices of the heart, with or without heat or fire). Points are then chosen to nourish the heart, calm the shen, and/or clear heart, drain fire, transform phlegm, and open the orifices, as needed.

Vacuity and Repletion

The way in which liver depression qi stagnation and shen disturbance combine with, exacerbate, or precipitate tendencies towards vacuity of qi–yang and/or blood–yin is analyzed. Additionally, the extent to which dampness and phlegm accumulate (repletion of yin), and the extent to which yang becomes replete (hyperactive liver yang, liver fire, or vacuity heart), is also evaluated. Points are then chosen to supplement vacuity of qi–yang and/or yin–blood, and/or to transform dampness and phlegm, clear heat, drain fire, etc., in order to regulate yin and yang based on the presenting signs and symptoms.

Viscera and Bowels

The involvement and role of each viscus and bowel and the functional interactions among them are analyzed. On one hand, special attention is paid to how the mechanisms of depression affect each one of their functions. On the other hand, the extent to which their dysfunction precipitates this particular depression episode is also determined.

Channels and Network Vessels

The 12 regular channels plus du mai, ren mai, and chong mai are the only channels used in our protocol. To regulate the flow of qi, stimulate brain function, and clear the heart's orifices, the use of points along the du channel is emphasized. To help refine point selection, the use of palpation of both the channels and the abdominal area is encouraged. Additionally, the concept of the six great units as constitutional predispositions (based on Yves Requena's eight diatheses (Requena 1986) has been used as a diagnostic tool; the six great units have also been used as guidelines for effective point combinations.

The Five Phases

The precipitating factors, the nature of the depressive episode, and the constitutional predisposition of the patient are analyzed by using the five phases as a framework. Primarily, Denmei's (1990) concept of constitutional types as predisposing factors, Beinfield & Korngold's (1991) five phases as types, and the classic five phases correspondences (Maciocia 1989) have been used.

In our protocol, the last two theories have been used exclusively to refine our understanding of the constitutional tendencies of each individual. These theories are used in order to design more effectively a treatment strategy that would address both circumstantial manifestations and trait tendencies. We believe that by using the five phases and the six units extensively as reframing tools, in both assessment and patient education, we gain the ability to capture the complexity of interaction between trait and circumstantial tendencies, between the branch and the root.

It would be well beyond the scope of this manual to present in detail any of those two theories. The interested reader is invited to consult the sources cited in the References for an indepth overview of the use of the six units and the five phases in diagnosis.

Implementation of the Assessment Framework

After using conventional Western assessment techniques to diagnose major depression and to exclude other relevant conditions, we perform a differential diagnosis on all participants entering treatment. The differential diagnosis is accomplished by using the traditional method of the four evaluations (Kaptchuk 1983, Maciocia 1989). The basic procedure is as follows.

Questioning

First, a questionnaire is administered (see Appendix A). In the first section, we ask about the precipitating factors, previous history of depression, and the person's unique experience of being depressed. We aim at getting a clear sense of the person's constitutional tendencies, the psychosocial nature of their depression, and how their lifestyle has influenced their health. It is in this section that we make the most use of the six great units, the five phases, and the eight principles, to understand constitutional tendencies. In the second section of the questionnaire, we focus on differentiating the symptom criteria for major depressive episode (DSM-IV) on the basis of our theoretical framework; special attention is paid to how the symptom criteria correspond to liver depression, qi stagnation, shen disturbance, and vacuity or repletion of yin and yang (see Table 3.1). During the interview, the assessors probe the questions in detail, to differentiate disease mechanisms and pattern combinations clearly. For women, we take an indepth gynecological history, including menstrual cycles, pregnancies, etc. We conclude by inquiring about the emotional nature of the patient's complaints and the current specific manifestations of the depression.

Palpation

Pulses are taken in the traditional fashion, as detailed in *The Secret of Chinese Pulse Diagnosis* (Flaws 1995). The main pulse definitions employed can be found in Appendix B. Additional information on pulse diagnosis is taken from Kaptchuk (1983) and Maciocia (1989).

Although not officially part of our research protocol, clinically we have found it helpful to perform abdominal palpation following the traditional Japanese system. We base our findings on Denmai's (1990) *Introduction to Meridian Therapy* (1990), Matsumoto & Birch's (1988) *Hara Diagnosis: Reflections on the Sea*, and Seem's (1990) *Acupuncture Imaging*. We also encourage palpation of the channel pathways and zones when making the final selection of points.

Observation, Listening/Smelling

Assessment of the tongue is based on *Tongue Diagnosis in Chinese Medicine* (Maciocia 1987). We follow traditional observation of the patient's demeanor and features (face color, eye expression, *shen*, etc.).

Synopsis

We determine the pattern(s), treatment principles, and treatment strategy by emphasizing differentiation of signs and symptoms, and pulse and tongue evaluation, as traditionally performed in the eight principles model. We begin with the premise that liver depression qi stagnation and an inability of the heart to store the *shen* properly underlie the disharmony in most cases. We determine to what extent this is true and explore whether the stagnation is affecting other viscera, and whether the shen disturbance is due to vacuity or repletion disease mechanisms. Additionally, based on the information gathered, we assess to what extent the pattern is characterized by yang features (psychomotor agitation, dream-disturbed sleep, and irritability) and develops along the yin vacuity–yang repletion continuum. Similarly, we determine the extent to which the pattern is characterized by yin features (psychomotor retardation, fatigue, hypersomnia) and develops along a vacuity of qi–yang/repletion of yin continuum (see Table 3.1). The involvement of each viscus and bowel is analyzed as well.

The following is a summary of the approach:

1. The acupuncturist performs a Chinese Medicine assessment using the intake form (provided in Appendix A) as a guide to gather information about the signs and symptoms, inquiring verbally about problem areas.

2. Tongue and pulse evaluation helps determine the disease mechanisms and pattern(s) involved. (Abdominal palpation and assessment of the channels assist in focusing the diagnosis.)

3. The acupuncturist arrives at a set of treatment principles to address the pattern or combination of patterns, by focusing on four features:

   a. liver depression qi stagnation

   b. shen disturbance due to either vacuity or repletion disease mechanisms, or both

   c. vacuity of qi–yang and/or (repletion) accumulation of dampness/phlegm

   d. vacuity of yin–blood and/or (repletion) hyperactivity of heat/fire.

4. Points are selected as detailed in the section Strategies and techniques.

TABLE 5.1A	Summary table for patterns				
Stagnation	**Shen disturbance**	**Qi/yang vacuity**	**Yin repletion: dampness and phlegm**	**Blood/ yin vacuity**	**Yang repletion and vacuity heat**

Stagnation	Shen disturbance	Qi/yang vacuity	Yin repletion: dampness and phlegm	Blood/ yin vacuity	Yang repletion and vacuity heat
Liver qi stagnation: chest, lateral costal, breast and abdominal distension and oppression; nausea, sensation of lump in the throat, premenstrual tension; moodiness, irritability. If severe, insomnia *Pulse:* wiry *Tongue:* normal or slightly dark, thin coating	**Vacuity** *Vacuity (qi/blood):* heart palpitations, anxiety, poor memory, dizziness, easily startled *Heart blood vacuity:* insomnia with difficulty falling asleep *Pulse:* fine, maybe choppy *Tongue:* pale, thin coat Depression with fatigue, confusion, lack of concentration	*Spleen qi vacuity.* lethargy, lack of appetite, no strength in the extremities, loose stools *Pulse:* relaxed, or soggy and weak *Tongue:* pale, swollen with thin white coating	*Spleen vacuity, dampness accumulating:* edema, chest and epigastric fullness and oppression, nausea, diarrhea *Pulse:* soggy, fine, or wiry fine; or slippery and relaxed *Tongue:* swollen pale, with teeth marks on the edges, and a thin, slimy, white coat	*Liver blood vacuity:* dizziness, numbness in limbs, insomnia, (difficulty falling asleep), blurred vision, scanty menses, dull pale complexion *Pulse:* fine, wiry, maybe choppy *Tongue:* pale, thin coating. Depression with fatigue, no sense of direction, afraid of making decisions	*Liver qi stagnation transforming into heat:* see qi stagnation *Hyperactive liver yang:* yang counterflows upwards and combines with symptoms of deficiency and cold below: headache, dizziness, vertigo, insomnia, irritability *Pulse:* wiry, rapid *Tongue:* red
Liver depression transforms heat: irascibility, easy anger, chest oppression, heart vexation, restlessness, insomnia, excessive dreams, bitter taste in the mouth, acne, thirst, constipation, early or excessive menstruation *Pulse:* wiry and rapid *Tongue:* dark red or dark and swollen edges with a thin, yellow coat	With Heart qi vacuity: shortness of breath, worst upon exertion *Pulse:* also weak *Heart yin vacuity:* insomnia with difficulty staying asleep, anxiety worst in the evening, fidgety *Pulse:* rapid, thin or floating, vacuous *Tongue:* red/redder tip, no coating	*Lu qi vacuity:* shortness of breath, spontaneous perspiration, cough on exertion *Pulse:* faint or vacuous and large *Tongue:* pale, swollen with thin, white coating	*Phlegm confounding the heart:* dullness of thought, fuzzy head, confusion, dizziness. Tired, subdued, quiet; tendency towards obsessive thinking, rumination *Pulse:* slippery, soggy *Tongue:* swollen body with a sticky white coating	*Liver yin vacuity:* deep depression, lack of purpose, confusion about aims and objectives, poor memory, dry eyes, skin, hair *Kidney yin vacuity:* great exhaustion, lack of will power and drive, decrease mental capacities and memory	*Liver fire flaming upward:* aggression, violent outburst of anger, headache, later costal pain, bitter taste in the mouth *Pulse:* rapid, forceful, slippery, wiry *Tongue:* red with slimy yellow coating
Qi stagnation affecting the heart/lung: oppression/tightness in the chest, sighing, palpitations, breathlessness, weepiness, easily affected by others' problems. Pale complexion *Pulse:* weak in the cun position, no wave *Note:* In the later stages stagnation can combine with dampness, phlegm, stasis of blood or fire	With vacuity heat: symptoms are more pronounced, sleep disturbance is extreme, aggressive, impatient **Repletion** *Stagnation: as in qi:* stagnation affecting the heart/lung *Depressive heat affecting the heart/lung* (see Liver depression transforms heat) *Heart fire:* Agitation, insomnia, excessive and disturbing dreams, racing heart *Pulse:* rapid, wiry, thready, if combined with vacuity; if combined with repletion, surging or slippery *Tongue:* red or red tip, ulcerated	*Spleen yang vacuity:* edema, fatigue after eating, cold body, chilled extremities *Pulse:* weak, deep, slow *Tongue:* swollen, pale, thin, white coating *Kidney qi vacuity:* low back and knee sore and weak, frequent urination, nocturia, loss of hair, low libido *Pulse:* deep, weak *Tongue:* pale red *With kidney yang vacuity:* pronounced sensitivity to cold	*Heart vacuity, gall bladder timidity:* difficulty making decisions, lack of courage and direction, easily startled, suceptibility to fright and fear *Pulse:* vacuous, weak *Tongue:* pale moist *Phlegm dampness obstruction and stagnation:* plum-pit qi, postnasal drip, excessive phlegm, fatigue, hypersomnia, confusion, rumination *Pulse:* wiry/slippery *Tongue:* slimy, white *Phlegm/fire:* agitation, easy anger, incessant talking, insomnia, bitter taste in the mouth, chest oppression, excess phlegm, constipation *Pulse:* rapid, wiry, large, slippery *Tongue:* red with thick yellow coat	*For yin vacuity in any of the three viscera:* *Pulse:* floating, empty *Tongue:* red, no coat	*Yin vacuity, fire effulgence:* from yin and blood vacuity, it agitates the shen and causes severe anxiety, insomnia, agitation, night sweats, afternoon fevers, heat in the palms, the soles, and the center of the chest. heart palpitations, malar flush *Pulse:* rapid, floating, empty *Tongue:* red, no coating, crack center, redder tip *Spleen vacuity giving rise to fire:* combination of qi/ yang vacuity, damp heat in lower heater and heat repletion in the upper heater symptoms *Pulse:* floating, large, slippery *Tongue:* swollen, red tip, yellow coat

TABLE 5.1B	Summary table for treatment principles				
Stagnation	**Shen disturbance**	**Qi/yang vacuity**	**Yin repletion: dampness and phlegm**	**Blood/ yin vacuity**	**Yang repletion and vacuity heat**
Liver depression, qi stagnation: course the liver, rectify the qi, and resolve depression	**Vacuity** *Vacuity qi and blood:* Nourish the heart, calm the spirit (boost the qi and supplement the blood)	*Qi vacuity:* in general, boost the qi *Spleen qi vacuity:* in addition, fortify the spleen	*Spleen vacuity, dampness accumulating:* fortify the spleen and transform dampness	*Liver blood vacuity:* nourish the liver and supplement the blood	*Liver qi stagnation transforms heat:* see under qi stagnation
Liver depression transforms heat: in addition to above, clear heat	*Deficient heart yin:* enrich yin, settle the heart and calm the spirit	*Lung qi vacuity:* in addition, fortify the lungs	*Phlegam dampness confounding the heart:* transform dampness, eliminate phlegm, open the orifices of the heart	*Liver yin vacuity:* nourish the liver, enrich yin, settle the hun, and quiet the spirit	*Hyperactive liver yang:* pacify the liver, subdue rebellious yang, clear heat, supplement and boost the liver and kidney
Qi stagnation affecting the heart/lung: in addition, stimulate the descending of heart and lung qi	*With vacuity heat:* in addition, clear vacuity heat	*Spleen yang vacuity:* in addition, warm yang	*Heart vacuity, gall bladder timidity:* warm the gall bladder, nourish the heart, quiet the spirit	*Lung yin vacuity:* enrich yin and moisten the lung	*Liver fire flaming upward:* clear the liver and drain fire, quiet the spirit, and settle the hun
	Repletion *Stagnation:* as in qi stagnation affecting the heart/lung	*Kidney qi vacuity:* in addition, supplement the kidney	*Phelgm dampness obstruction and stagnation:* transform phlegm, disinhibit qi, and resolve depression	*Kidney yin vacuity:* supplement the kidney and enrich yin	*Vacuity heat:* enrich, yin, clear heat or drain fire, settle the heart, and calm the spirit
	Depressive heart: as in liver depression, transformative heat	*Kidney yang vacuity:* in addition, warm kidney yang			
	Heart fire: harmonize the heart, clear heat, drain fire, and settle the spirit		*Phlegm/fire:* in addition, clear the liver and drain fire		*Spleen vacuity fire:* supplement spleen, transform dampness, clear heat

TABLE 5.1C	Summary table for points				
Stagnation	**Shen disturbance**	**Qi/yang vacuity**	**Yin repletion: dampness and phlegm**	**Blood/ yin vacuity**	**Yang repletion and vacuity heat**
Points for each pattern *General stagnation:* Lv 3, LI 4	**Vacuity**	*Spleen qi vacuity:* UB 20, UB 21, UB 49, Ren 4, Ren 6, St 36, Sp 3, Ren 12	*Spleen vacuity, dampness accumulating:* add Sp 5, Ren 9, Sp 9 to spleen vacuity points	*Liver blood vacuity:* UB 17, UB 18, UB 20, Ub 47, Lv 8	*Liver qi stagnation transforms heat:* see under Qi stagnation
Liver depression, qi stagnation: Lv 14, UB 18	**Vacuity in general** UB 15, UB 44, Ren 14, Ht 7, P 6 *In addition use: Heart blood vacuity:* Ren 4, St 36, Sp 6, Sp 4	*Lu qi vacuity:* UB 13, Lu 1, Lu 7, Lu 9, UB 42	*Phlegm confounding the heart:* add St 40, LI 4 to points under spleen vacuity (above), dampness accumulating (above)	*Liver yin vacuity:* add UB 23, UB 52, Kd 3, Kd 6, Kd 10	*Hyperactive liver yang:* GB 20, Lv 2, Lv 3, LI 11, GB 20, Yintang
Liver depression transforms heat: Add Lv 2, LI 11, P 7 to points that regulate liver depression, qi stagnation	*Heart qi vacuity:* Ren 4, St 36, Sp 6, Sp 4 *Heart yin vacuity:* P 7, Kd 6, Kd 3, Kd 10, Sp 6, Ht 7	*Spleen yang vacuity:* same as spleen qi deficiency above (moxa is applicable)	*Heart vacuity, gallbladder timidity:* GB 40, Ht 7	*Kidney yin vacuity:* UB 23, UB 57, Kd 3, Kd 6, Kd 10, Sp 6, Kd 22, Kd 27 *Lung yin vacuity:*	*Liver fire flaming upward:* Lv 2, Lv 3, UB 18, Sp 6, GB 15, Du 24 and GB 13, Ht 7, P 7
Qi stagnation affecting the heart/lung: Lu 7, P 6, Ht 7, Ren 17, Sp 21, Ren 15	*With vacuity heat:* Ht 6 **Repletion** *Depressive heat:* as for transforms heat	*Kidney qi vacuity:* UB 23, UB 52, Ren 6, Kd 3, Kd 7, Du 4 *Kidney yang vacuity:* same as kidney qi deficiency above (moxa is applicable)	*Phlegm dampness obstruction and stagnation:* to points above add Ren 17, Ren 12, Sp 21, GB 17, GB 18	UB 13, UB 42, Lu 7, Sp 6	*Vacuity heat:* add to points that nourish yin: Kd 2 with Lv 3, Ht 6 *Spleen vacuity fire:* Ren 4, Ren 6, Ren 15, UB 20, UB 23, Sp 9, Sp 6, Ht 5
	Qi stagnation affecting the heart (and lung): see under qi stagnation				

cont.

cont.

Stagnation	Shen disturbance	Qi/yang vacuity	Yin repletion: dampness and phlegm	Blood/ yin vacuity	Yang repletion and vacuity heat
			Phlegm fire: same as above plus points to clear the liver and transform fire: Lv 2, LI 11, Ht 8, GB 15		
	Heart fire: Ht 8, GB 15				

Source: Flaws & Finney (1996), Maciocia (1994), with permission.

TABLE 5.1D	*Frequently used points organized by meridian or channel*

Outer urinary bladder	Heart	Pericardium	Kidney	Small intestine	Gall bladder	Lung	RenMo (conception vessel)	DuMo (governing vessel)
UB 42, 44, 47, 49, 52	Ht 7, 6, 8	P 7, 6	Kd 9	SI 5, 3	GB 13, 15, 17, 18, 40	Lu 7	Ren 15, 4	Du 18, 19, 20, 21, 24

Source: Flaws & Finney (1996), Maciocia (1994), with permission.

TABLE 5.2	*Auricular points commonly used in the depression protocol*

No.	Name	Location	Function
1	Master point zero	Located in a notch, at the beginning of the helix root	Brings the whole body into homeostatic balance; facilitates willpower
2	Shenmen	Located medial to the apex of the triangular fossa	Alleviates pain, tension, anxiety, and depression
3	Sympathetic tone	Located at the medial end of the inferior crus, covered by the helix junction above it	Balances sympathetic nervous system activity; improves vascular circulation
4	Cheerfulness	Located in the lobe, below the antitragal incisure	Relieves depression
5	Excitement	Located in the wall of the antitragus	Relieves hypersomnia and depression
6	Master cerebral point	Located where the medial lobe joins the face	Diminishes anxiety, worry, obsessive–compulsive disorders, psychosomatic disorders, and chronic pain
7	Master oscillation point	Located on the subtragus, on the internal side of the inferior knob	Balances the left and right cerebral hemispheres, corrects problems of laterality
8	Sleep disorders 1	Located in the scaphoid fossa	Relieves insomnia, nervousness.
9	Sleep disorders 2	Located on the internal helix	Relieves insomnia, sleep difficulties, nervous dreams, inability to dream

Source: Oleson (1992).

<table>
<tr><td>

6

</td><td>

Case Studies

</td></tr>
</table>

INTRODUCTION

To provide an illustration of how the framework applies to clients who have been treated, and to demonstrate the integration of the Western and Chinese Medicine perspective, we provide two case histories of individuals who were treated with acupuncture as part of our research protocol, and who responded favorably to treatment. Furthermore, to help illustrate the limitations of how well the framework applies to clients who have been treated, an additional two case histories are provided of individuals who were treated with acupuncture, but who did not respond fully during the course of the research protocol. All four cases met DSM-IV criteria for major depression but, as indicated below, there were many differences in how their depression presented.

In gaging the success of the acupuncture treatment, several measures are typically used in research studies of depression. The main measure is an interview, the Hamilton Depression Rating Scale (HRSD) (Hamilton 1967). This clinician-administered interview provides ratings of the severity of depression, symptom by symptom (e.g. for sleep disturbance, for mood disturbance, etc.). Scores are then totaled to yield a summary score of the severity of a person's depression. To enter most treatment studies of depression, individuals must have HRSD scores greater than 14. Scores close to 14 would be considered mild depression, whereas scores above 20 indicate moderate to severe depression.

TANYA

Tanya was 48 years old when she began the study. She had experienced several depressive episodes, the first one at age 34 years. She had a history of chronic depression, although the current episode was not chronic. Tanya had previously received psychotherapy and medication for her depression. Just before the beginning of the study, she had been taking L-tryptophan for 2.5 years under the care of her naturopathic physician. Without this supplement, Tanya felt a marked exacerbation of her symptoms and increased sensitivity. The current episode was triggered by difficulties with her present boyfriend; she had been married and divorced several times and believed that her tendency towards depression had always been tied to fear of abandonment and difficulties in her interpersonal relationships. She had also recently experienced numerous significant losses. As a condition of entry into the study, Tanya discontinued the use of L-tryptophan.

Western Assessment

Tanya experienced both depressed mood and anhedonia. In addition, she had a decreased appetite, as well as insomnia with difficulty going back to sleep, especially in the early morning. She also reported restlessness and agitation, a low sense of self-esteem, and thoughts about suicide that did not involve any active wish to die or plan to do so. At the beginning of the study her HRSD score was 23 (moderate depression).

Chinese Medicine Assessment

Tanya described her depression as a profound sense of sadness and hopelessness about her inability to change anything in her life; she felt defeated and that she lacked any reason to be around. She felt indecisive, insecure, aimless. She was frequently agitated, anxious, and tearful. Tanya was terrified of not measuring up to people's expectations and, therefore, she felt incapable of doing anything on her own. In addition to her symptoms of depression, Tanya suffered from chronic muscle pain syndrome, environmental sensitivities, and hyperreactivity to external stimuli. Tanya craved sweets and felt a worsening of her symptoms if she ate sugar. She also experienced heaviness in her limbs, retained water in her abdomen and hands, and had excessive white vaginal discharge and itchiness.

Upon examination Tanya's pulse was found to be surging in the second position on the right, wiry and slightly choppy in the first position on both sides, and vacuous and soft in the third position. Her tongue (Fig. 6.1) was generally swollen with scalloped edges, dark, and trembling; it had a white coating, thicker at the back; it was especially swollen along an indentation in the center, and was slightly deviated to the left. Tanya's pattern differentiation encompasses the complex yin fire scenario described in Chapters 3 and 5. She presented a combination of: spleen qi–kidney yang vacuity, liver blood–kidney yin vacuity, depressive heat (affecting heart and lungs), and dampness accumulation. Heat stemming from liver depression, spleen vacuity, and kidney vacuity were agitating the *shen* or spirit. Secondarily, phlegm arising from the dampness generated by spleen vacuity was confounding the orifices of the heart. The treatment principles were to supplement the spleen and nourish the kidney, transform dampness and phlegm, clear heat, rectify the qi, and relieve depression. A treatment combination sample included the following points: Sp 4 left, P 6 right, Lv 3 left, Sp 6 bilateral, Kd 9 right, Ht 5 left, Ren 4, Du 24, and GB 13.

Outcome

At the completion of the study, Tanya expressed feeling open to taking risks, free of fear and negative thinking, trustful of herself and others, hopeful about the future, capable of standing on her own two feet, and optimistic. Additionally she experienced a significant reduction of her physical symptoms. She was practically free of depressive symptoms; her HRSD score was only 2 and she no longer met criteria for depression according to DSM-IV.

KAREN

Karen was 64 years old when she began the study. She had a history of chronic depression, one of her episodes lasted 3 consecutive years; she had experienced numerous episodes since her early teens. In the last 4 years she experienced moderate to severe depression, resulting from limited activity caused by degenerative back disease. In the last couple of years her depression had become severe owing to the loss of several close loved ones over a short period of time. Before the beginning of the study she had been taking St John's wort to treat her depression, but stopped 2 weeks before being interviewed to meet eligibility for the study.

Western Assessment

Karen described her depression as having a low but persistent level of moodiness, frequent crying and irritability, chronic fatigue, lack of energy, difficulty sleeping, frequent awakening during the night, and difficulty returning to sleep. Additionally, she experienced increased appetite and a lack of self-esteem. When she began the study her HRSD score was 23 (moderate depression).

Chinese Medicine Assessment

Karen reported cravings for sweets, chronic lower backache, sinus congestion, and postnasal drip. She had received estrogen replacement therapy since the age of 42 years, and had continued having menstrual cycles until the last couple of years. She had a history of drinking several cups of coffee per day, of smoking marijuana regularly, and of drinking grain alcohol regularly, in moderation. (Karen did not meet DSM-IV criteria, however, for alcohol abuse or dependence.) After examination, Karen's pulse was found to be deep, forceless, and slightly choppy. Her tongue (Fig. 6.2) was very swollen, purple-pale, trembling, with a pronounced crack on the tip, darker sides and tip, and a wet thin coat. Karen's pattern differentiation was liver stasis and stagnation, spleen–heart dual vacuity, kidney yin and yang dual vacuity with vacuity heat, and dampness accumulation due to spleen vacuity. Shen disturbance was due to liver depression and stasis, and due to vacuity heat agitating the spirit.

The treatment principles were to course the liver and rectify the qi, transform stasis, supplement the spleen and nourish the heart, enrich yin, clear heat, calm the *shen*, and settle the hun. A sample of a treatment plan included the following points: UB 44, UB 47, and UB 52 (leaving needles in for 10 minutes only), UB 23, KD 3 bilateral, Ht 6 right.

Outcome

At the end of the study, Karen expressed not having felt so good for many years; her outlook in life was much better, she felt optimistic and confident, and looked forward to every day and the future. Karen felt energetic and stronger; her sleep improved, although she still met criteria for insomnia. At the end of the study, Karen's HRSD score was 2, and she no longer met criteria for depression according to DSM-IV.

FRANCESCA

Francesca was 33 years old when she began the study. She had experienced depression several times in the past, but had no history of chronic depression. Her current episode appeared to begin 6 years ago, but had been punctuated by periods of remission that were at least 2 months in duration. Francesca was unsure what precipitated the onset, but thought it was related to the birth of her son. She had tried antidepressants in the past and found fluoxetine (Prozac) effective. She had also used St John's wort, and felt it had helped somewhat, but she still felt depressed.

Western Assessment

Francesca described her depression as being sad and irritable all the time, having no interest or energy for anything, and feeling bored with everything. She also gained 27 lbs in 9 months, felt worthless, and could not make decisions. Her husband had died about 6 months before she entered the study, and a few months after that she discontinued Prozac. The depression preceded her husband's death, but became worse after it. Her HRSD score was 22 (moderate depression) at the beginning of the study.

Chinese Medicine Assessment

In addition to the characteristic depression symptoms noted above, Francesca suffered from restless leg syndrome, which was slightly alleviated by walking, especially on a cold surface, and she experienced irritable bowels and constipation. Premenstrually, she retained water, had breast distension, had diffuse pain in the lower back and hips, and increased irritability with violent outbursts of anger. Her menstrual flow had become heavier and had dark clots in it.

The onset of Francesca's depression following the birth of her son stresses the importance of looking at the details of her pregnancy and labor. She had had a good pregnancy and birth, but it was a time of a lot of stress in her life. She became very sad and irritable postpartum; she breastfed for 8 months and her menstruation returned 2 months later.

In general, Francesca's sleep was restless, and she woke up frequently throughout the night. Her pulse was vacuous and soggy in the second position on the right, fine and wiry in the second position on the left, and alternated between having no wave and being wiry in the first position on both hands. Her tongue (Fig. 6.3) was slightly swollen around the edges, but thin, palish with redder sides, and had a slightly wet, thin coating.

Francesca's pattern differentiation was depressive heat affecting the heart and lung, heart–spleen dual vacuity, some kidney vacuity, and slight blood stasis. Depressive heat and heart blood vacuity were affecting the heart's ability to house the *shen*; additionally, there was some phlegm confounding the orifices of the heart as a result of spleen qi vacuity. The treatment principles were to course the liver and rectify the qi (this would clear heat on its own), assist the descending of lung qi, boost qi and blood, supplement the spleen and heart; secondarily the principles were to transform dampness, clear phlegm, and open the heart's orifices. A sample treatment plan involved the following points: Lv 3 on the right, P 6 on the left, Sp 21 bilateral, Ren 4, Kd 3 bilateral, Lu 7 on the right, GB 18 bilateral.

Outcome

Francesca experienced some improvement: her depressive symptoms were not as frequent or intense, her appetite and her energy had returned to normal, and she became a bit more patient; her HRSD score was 12. She still felt depressed more days than not, however, thought that she would be better off dead, and continued to have decreased interest in activities. Francesca decided that acupuncture was not helping her to improve as much as she wished and dropped out of the study after 12 weeks of treatment. She believed that her depression was negatively affecting her relationship with her son, and decided to seek another type of treatment. Francesca no longer met full DSM-IV criteria for depression at the end of the study. She still had significant symptoms of depression when she discontinued treatment; therefore her treatment was considered to be unsuccessful.

Commentary

Francesca had several features that could be considered poor prognostic signs. From the Western perspective, although her current episode was not chronic by virtue of having discrete periods of remission, over the last 6 years she had a fairly chronic history. Additionally, her depression was exacerbated by bereavement and many psychosocial stressors.

From the perspective of Chinese Medicine, the fact that the onset of her depression seemed to coincide with the birth of her son indicated that the spleen–heart dual vacuity was likely the result of high levels of stress, confounded by the natural changes in her body due to pregnancy. During pregnancy, the demand on the spleen to generate qi and blood is increased; if, in addition, liver depression qi stagnation further weakens the spleen, both qi and blood vacuity may ensue. Furthermore, severe or prolonged spleen qi vacuity often leads to kidney vacuity. Although the depression preceded her husband's death, the loss of her spouse and the other dramatic changes that followed in her life further exacerbated damage to the heart by liver depression. A longer course of treatment, and acupuncture coupled with psychotherapy, may have yielded better results for Francesca.

TIM

Tim was 39 when he started the study. He had experienced a chronic low-level depression for most of his life (dysthymia), interspersed with numerous major depressive episodes. Tim first sought treatment for depression at around age 20 years; he had received both psychotherapy and antidepressant medication for depression in the past, but had not found either very helpful. Although he had experienced several periods of normal mood for several months at a time, he reported having had relatively few periods when he actually felt good. The current major depressive episode had lasted for 5 months; it was precipitated by difficulty finding employment after returning from living abroad, and by the breakup of a relationship.

Western Assessment

Tim did not experience any interest or pleasure in any activities; he felt worthless, could not make decisions, had difficulty concentrating, and experienced frequent thoughts of suicide that did not involve any active wish to die or plan to do so. He had irritability, insomnia with restless sleep, and tendency to ruminate; in addition, he frequently felt agitated and anxious. At the beginning of the study his HRSD score was 28 (moderate to severe depression).

Chinese Medicine Assessment

Tim described his depression as having no goals or direction in life, and feeling fearful, oppressed, unmotivated, lethargic, and hopeless. In addition to the symptoms specific to depression, Tim suffered from sinus headaches that were worst in the mornings and were exacerbated by humid weather and by eating greasy, fatty foods and eggs; he experienced relief from his headaches by drinking coffee. Tim also suffered from chronic lower backache due to a congenital problem and had cystic acne. Tim was a habitual marijuana smoker, and described the effects of cannabis on his depression as helping him not to focus on his problems. (Tim did not meet DSM-IV criteria, however, for substance abuse or dependence.)

Upon examination, it was found that Tim's pulse varied frequently in speed and strength; it alternated between wiry and slippery, and vacuous and soggy, especially in the second position. The third position was vacuous, at times floating, but mostly deep. His tongue (Fig. 6.4) was swollen with scalloped edges, dark with a purplish hue, trembling, and showed a deep center crack that reached almost to the tip, as well as red spots on the tip and sides. His tongue had a thin, white, and slightly frothy coating, which was thicker and slightly grayish in the back.

The Chinese pattern differentiation was liver depression transforming into heat, with underlying kidney yang vacuity and spleen qi vacuity. Shen disturbance was due to phlegm confounding the orifices of the heart, and to depressive heat agitating the spirit. Tim's long history of depression in the context of the other signs and symptoms indicated constitutional kidney yang vacuity underlining the acute episodes, as well as an element of blood stasis. The treatment principles were to course the liver and rectify the qi, clear heat, transform phlegm, open the heart's orifices, calm the spirit, supplement the spleen, and fortify the kidney. A sample treatment included the following points: Lv 3 bilateral, LI 4 right, P 6 on the left, St 40 and Kd 3 bilateral, Ren 15, Ht 5 left, GB 15 bilateral.

Outcome

At the completion of the study, Tim still felt depressed and did not think that any significant changes had taken place. Upon questioning, he mentioned a lessening of suicidal ideation, a decrease of self-doubt and rumination, and an improved ability to make decisions. He had some relief of his sense of hopelessness and felt more capable of helping himself. Tim was able to carry through a daily routine of exercise and relaxation, experienced improvement in his lower backache, and had substantially decreased his use of marijuana and alcohol. There was some improvement in his energy level, headaches, and sinus congestion. Shortly after completion of the study, Tim embarked himself in a new venture, and moved to a new town. His HRSD score, however, was 27 (moderate to severe depression), which indicated virtually no change in his depression.

Commentary

Tim had several features that could have contributed to his poor treatment response. From the Western perspective, he had a history of dysthymia and chronic depression. Although his current episode was not chronic by virtue of having experienced a discrete period of remission, in general he had a decidedly chronic history. In reviewing his case, he meets for the proposed set of diagnostic criteria for depressive personality disorder (DSM-IV, p. 733).

From the Chinese Medicine perspective, the small changes that Tim had experienced indicated a positive sign towards progress. Nevertheless, his symptom picture highlighted long-standing and constitutional vacuity, significant phlegm dampness obstruction and stagnation, and blood stasis. These three factors render short-term treatment by acupuncture alone insufficient. From the perspective of Chinese Medicine, the consistent use of Chinese herbal medicine in conjunction with acupuncture could assist in readdressing Tim's constitutional vacuity. Dietary and lifestyle changes directed at decreasing phlegm dampness obstruction and stagnation would potentiate the effect of acupuncture (Schnyer & Flaws 1998).

7 Research Considerations

INTRODUCTION

How do we know that a treatment works? This simple question is deceptively complex. When we observe that someone's symptoms disappear after receiving a particular treatment, we cannot unambiguously assume that the treatment itself was responsible for the changes we observed. For any client, there will be a wide range of potentially therapeutic factors, some part of the treatment setting and many outside of the treatment setting, that may influence the outcome. Moreover, even within the treatment setting, it can be quite difficult to specify just what components of a treatment are considered the essential or active components.

Treatment research seeks to determine not only whether treatments work, but also what particular factors are responsible for creating change. It is tempting to overlook these issues in everyday practice, as it may not seem relevant to know precisely what factors prompted a client to improve, as long as there was significant improvement. On the other hand, good clinical practice can benefit from the same type of careful observation as that seen in research trials. Moreover, the clinical practitioner can integrate new research findings into practice if he or she is equipped to evaluate the research literature carefully. This chapter will therefore provide an overview of research designs

Parts of this chapter appear in Schnyer & Allen (2001) and are included here with the permission of the publisher, WB Saunders.

and the questions that each can address. Additionally, specific issues related to designing acupuncture trials will be highlighted.

RESEARCH QUESTIONS: EFFECTIVENESS AND EFFICACY

There have been relatively few well-controlled trials of the efficacy of acupuncture in the treatment of depression. Although myriad clinical observations and a few research studies suggest that acupuncture is helpful (i.e. effective) in alleviating depressive symptoms, very few studies have addressed the more specific scientific question of whether the particular acupuncture points are critical in creating improvement in depression (i.e. efficacy). Studies of the *effectiveness* of a treatment address merely whether it is helpful. By contrast, studies of the *efficacy* of a treatment address whether the treatment works for the reasons it is purported to work. There are many research designs that have been and can be utilized in acupuncture research (Hammerschlag 1998), but each is only suited to address particular questions and to provide certain kinds of information.

Chinese Medicine provides a very clear framework for understanding the diverse presentations of the symptoms of depression, and for providing individually tailored treatments to address each person's pattern configuration. This framework very clearly indicates that the particular points used, in the service of addressing the treatment principles, are the active 'ingredient' in the treatment package. While one study (Allen et al 1998, summarized later in this chapter) suggests that the particular points may in fact be the critical element that creates improvement for those with depression, there are many other factors that may also prove therapeutic to the depressed person who receives acupuncture. Such factors include, among others, making a commitment to a treatment program designed to alleviate one's depression, having a relationship with a caring and attentive healthcare professional, holding the belief that one is receiving an effective treatment, and deliberately breaking one's routine to keep regular appointments outside the home. These factors have often been termed 'nonspecific' factors (Arkowitz 1992, Grencavage et al 1993) because they characterize virtually any treatment program, and are specific to none. While such nonspecific factors can exert powerful therapeutic effects, it is incumbent on the researcher interested in efficacy to demonstrate that the treatment under study is effective above and beyond such nonspecific factors.

It is also worth noting that these nonspecific factors extend beyond the common conception of the placebo effect. The placebo effect is often defined as that portion of treatment response due to the mere belief that one is receiving treatment. Belief, however, is but one of the many factors other than the treatment that may result in improvement. The factors listed above, as well as others unique to any particular treatment milieu, constitute the many other *active* factors besides the client's belief that (s)he is receiving a good treatment. Adequate research designs control for not only the placebo effect of expectations, but also for the other nonspecific but active factors that may influence outcome.

Before suggesting a 'gold standard' for research designs, it is worth considering the merits and limitations of other research designs that have been used in acupuncture research and summarized recently (Ernst 1998, Hammerschlag 1998). These other designs include: (1) case studies and clinical observations of acupuncture, (2) acupuncture compared with waitlist controls, (3) acupuncture compared with placebo controls, (4) acupuncture compared with sham controls and yoked sham controls, (5) acupuncture compared with standard care, and (6) acupuncture plus standard care compared with standard care only.

TREATMENT STUDY DESIGNS

Clinical Observation and Case Studies

As a starting point, clinical observation and case studies are important in that they provide the rudimentary evidence to suggest that further study is warranted. On the other hand, clinical observation and case studies do not inform us as to *why* a treatment may appear to work. In such studies, treatment response may be due to the effect of acupuncture per se, or it may be the result of other therapeutic factors such as the provider–client relationship or the belief that one is receiving an effective treatment, among others. Moreover, such designs involve retrospective interpretations which make it likely that data will be incomplete, and that the sample may be unrepresentative (e.g. the treatment failures are less likely to be noted or become the focus of a case study). Case studies are an important starting point, but do not provide definitive data.

Waitlist Controls

Waitlist control studies are an extension of clinical observation and case studies. These studies, which pit acupuncture against time alone (i.e. while people await treatment), are an improvement over clinical observation and case studies in that they provide systematic observation of more clients, they are prospective and therefore not subject to retrospective reporting bias, and they involve randomization to treatment or waitlist so that the people receiving treatment and those receiving no treatment are likely to be comparable. This design, however, suffers from many of the shortcomings of the previous design, most notably that the design does not address what specifically is responsible for any observed treatment benefit in the treatment group; the treatment response may be due to the effect of acupuncture per se, or it may be the result of other therapeutic factors.

Placebo Controls

Placebo controls, which are extremely popular as controls in pharmaceutical trials, involve an inert treatment. In drug trials, this is typically a sugar (or other inactive) pill. In acupuncture research, however, placebo controls are considerably more difficult to implement. Since placebo trials are, in the ideal, supposed to provide a control for the expectation of improvement by both client and provider, neither must know that the placebo treatment is in fact inert. Examples for acupuncture research include the use of placebo needles that do not penetrate the skin (Streitberger & Kleinhenz 1998) or the use of inactive transcutaneous electrical nerve stimulation (TENS) (cf. Petrie & Hazleman 1986). While such innovative techniques may provide an excellent control in some cases, they do not allow a direct comparison to standard needling techniques, and may therefore be limited in their application. Moreover, they may not allow for a blinding of the treatment provider in all cases, which could result in greater improvement in the active versus the placebo treatment group as a result of the provider's expectations that the active treatment is more effective than the placebo treatment (Berman 1980).

Sham Controls

Sham controls involve invasive needling of 'inert' or 'invalid' acupuncture points, often adjacent to the points that are part of the active treatment. It is often thought that such studies provide a control for expectations by clients, for the general therapeutic milieu, and for non-specific physiological effects of needle insertion. On the other hand, this design is quite undesirable in that it is impossible to conduct a double-blind study (see below for more on the importance of double blinding). Because the treatment provider is not blind when providing sham treatment, the provider will necessarily hold the belief that the sham treatment is ineffective or, if the provider is also providing the active acupuncture treatment, will think that the sham is much less effective than the active treatment. Because provider expectations can have profound influences on outcome (Berman 1980), this design should be avoided, or treated solely as a preliminary investigation.

An improvement on the sham control design is the yoked sham control design. This procedure may have limited applicability, but has been useful for ear acupuncture protocols in the treatment of substance abuse (e.g. Bullock et al 1989). In this design, two clients are treated side by side: one client receives the genuine treatment points, while the other receives the sham points. Other than the points provided, the experience of the two clients should be virtually identical, assuming the practitioner does not make remarks specifically to one client and not to the other. Structuring the treatment milieu in this fashion discourages the unblinded practitioner from treating clients differently as a function of which treatment they are receiving. While not as desirable as the double-blind study discussed below, this design provides a reasonably good control for nonspecific therapeutic factors.

Comparison with Standard Care

This design compares acupuncture to a treatment that is currently the standard of care and that – ideally – has demonstrated efficacy in rigorous clinical trials. In such designs, the merit of acupuncture is assumed if the treatment response of those receiving acupuncture is comparable to that of clients receiving the standard treatment. Such a design is ideally undertaken only after a strict efficacy study (see below) has been conducted. Moreover, two caveats are worth noting. The first is a statistical point. The logic of statistical tests is that one always attempts to find a significant difference between groups. Statistical tests allow one to infer, provided there is a significant difference between groups, that the difference is unlikely to have occurred by chance or, more precisely, that such a difference between groups would have occurred by chance only 5% of the time. (If it would have occurred by chance only 5% of the time, then it is reasonable to assume that the difference did not occur by chance and is, therefore, due to the treatment.) On the other hand, the finding of no difference between treatment groups does not allow one to make a statistically supported conclusion that the treatments are equivalent. There are many reasons that statistical tests can fail to find a significant difference, including the lack of an adequate sample size, excessive variability among client outcomes, and, of course, the fact that the treatments may actually be comparable.

The second caveat with this design concerns the impact of the standard treatment. The impact of any treatment in research studies varies considerably, and even well-validated treatments can, in some studies, fail to provide much in the way of a sizable treatment gain. Simply showing that acupuncture does not differ from the standard of care may not necessarily indicate that either is any better than a suitable control, because it is possible in a particular trial using this design that the standard treatment performed more poorly than usual. Because of this latter caveat, it is often useful in designs that compare acupuncture with a standard of care also to include either a waitlist control or some form of placebo treatment as a third group. In fact, this can be quite a powerful design as the placebo can be designed with respect to the standard treatment, and not the acupuncture treatment – a considerably easier task in most cases. In this 'three-arm' design, the efficacy of acupuncture would be indicated by a finding that acupuncture produced a larger treatment response than the placebo, regardless of whether it differed from standard care. Of course a stronger finding would be that acupuncture not only produced greater treatment gains than placebo, but also provided treatment gains at least as large as standard care.

Acupuncture Plus Standard Care Versus Standard Care Only

This design attempts to see whether there is any incremental advantage to adding acupuncture to an established treatment regimen. In the simplest form, the design compares standard treatment plus acupuncture to standard treatment alone. Of course, such a design is confounded in that the former group receives considerably more attention and can hold expectations for considerably greater improvement than the latter group. On the other hand, in situations where efficacy studies of acupuncture have already been conducted, such a design can address the extent to which acupuncture may assist as a complementary treatment. A stronger design would involve a double-blind study in which standard treatment plus acupuncture was compared with standard treatment plus some other placebo treatment. The latter would involve similar time and attention and expectancy, but would lack efficacy. In such a design, the superiority of the former treatment over the latter would suggest that acupuncture could be an important complementary treatment to established treatments. The best and most powerful example of this is the recent study examining the addition of fish oil (versus the addition of the placebo of olive oil) to the standard care for manic depressive illness (Stoll et al 1999).

THE GOLD STANDARD IN EFFICACY DESIGNS

While each of the designs noted above can play an important role in investigating whether acupuncture has merit in the treatment of various conditions, there remains nonetheless a gold standard for establishing efficacy; that is, establishing that the pure effect of a treatment such as acupuncture – unconfounded by other therapeutic aspects of the treatment delivery – is sufficient to produce clinically significant gains.

Double-blind RCTs

In order to demonstrate such efficacy, the double-blind randomized control trial (RCT) is used. Only the RCT can provide rigorous scientific tests of the efficacy of any untested treatment, including alternative treatments. The first critical component of the RCT is that research participants are randomly chosen to receive one of two treatments that are identical in every respect *except* for the purported essential ingredient. Placebo-controlled drug studies are the best example of this principle. Clients in both groups receive identical looking pills and dosing schedules, with the only difference being the actual content of the pills. All other nonspecific factors, such as the nature of and quantity of contact with the treatment staff, are comparable between the groups. In order for the nature of the contact with the staff to be comparable, however, the second critical aspect of the RCT must be present: both the recipients and the providers of treatment must be blinded as to whether a particular treatment is hypothesized to be effective. If either recipients or providers were to discern which treatment was hypothesized to be more effective, this would change the nature of the relationship and the expectations regarding how effective the treatment would be. Such expectancies can exert powerful influences on treatment response; for example, placebo responses are about 75% as large as drug responses using Prozac to treat depression (Kirsch & Sapirstein 1998).

Issues in Blinding

Although the double-blind study is challenging to carry out, it is often assumed in double-blind research on mental disorders that the study is double blind in two senses. The first is that neither the client nor the person rating the outcome is aware of what treatment the client has been receiving. The second is that neither the client nor the provider of the treatment knows what treatment the client has received. So, in a sense, the gold standard for treatment should entail a triple-blind study, where neither client nor provider nor outcome assessor is aware of the treatment received by the client.

When it comes to conducting efficacy trials of acupuncture in Western cultures, blinding the client is relatively easy, as long as the client perceives some needling. Few individuals in Western society know where acupuncture points are located, much less which points might aid in their particular presentation of depression. It is much more difficult to blind the treatment provider. The use of inactive ('sham') acupuncture does not adequately blind the treatment provider, as the provider is fully aware of which treatments are valid and which are invalid. Such awareness will lead the provider to have a different expectation of outcome for sham versus active treatments. These expectations can, and should, be assessed in any efficacy study.

The thorny issue of blinding the acupuncture treatment provider is difficult, but not impossible, to resolve. As described elsewhere in this manual, the allopathic condition 'depression' can be seen as an imbalance in the person's pattern configuration and may be interpreted using different frameworks based on the Chinese Medicine model. And because treatments need to be tailored to each individual in order to provide the maximum benefit, any two depressed individuals are likely to receive rather different constellations of points in their treatment. Thus, if any acupuncture treatment provider were only to receive a set of points to administer, it would not be immediately obvious whether such points would be designed to address a pattern imbalance underlying a particular client's depression. Following this logic a bit further, it is therefore possible to separate two traditionally integrated functions of the acupuncturist treatment provider: assessment versus treatment. If assessors only served to conceptualize the treatment principles and devise the treatment strategy and associated points, and a different group of treating acupuncturists were provided with these points to administer to clients, then there would be a reasonable chance that these treating acupuncturists would be blind as to whether a treatment would be the most effective for a given client. Thus, while the providers would not be blind as to what points were used, they may well be blinded as to the particular intent of the treatment. This strategy presumes that two important restrictions are employed: (1) that the treating acupuncturists are prohibited from using assessment procedures (including the interview, palpation, taking of pulses, and examination of the tongue, and (2) that the treating acupuncturists are not fully aware of which theoretical framework (i.e. combination of filters) is being employed to conceptualize the client. While this strategy would not guarantee that the treating acupuncturist would remain blind, the effectiveness of this strategy in producing a double blind can be monitored by simply administering questionnaires that tap the expectancies and beliefs of the provider and recipient. This is the strategy we used in our pilot study (Allen et al 1998).

Treatment Fidelity

Implicit in the foregoing discussion is that any acupuncture treatment should be faithfully derived from the framework of Chinese Medicine. As Hammerschlag (1998) has pointed out, it is clearly inappropriate to implement an invariant treatment for all clients in a study based solely on Western biomedical diagnoses. Because there exists considerable heterogeneity – in Chinese Medicine terms – among those who share a common allopathic diagnosis, any single set of acupuncture points applied to all clients would be absurd from the perspective of Chinese Medicine. Instead, careful differential diagnosis from the perspective of Chinese Medicine is required to arrive at individually tailored treatments that Chinese Medicine would predict address the underlying pattern of imbalance. Such individual tailoring may seem at first glance to be in conflict with the scientific need to standardize the treatment approach, but it is possible to deliver manualized, replicable, and standardized treatments that are nonetheless tailored to each client on the basis of that client's pattern of disharmony. This manual was written with precisely this aim in mind.

Ethical Sensitivity

Many acupuncture practitioners and researchers have worried about whether various research designs are ethical, in that some may not necessarily provide a treatment known to be (or thought to be) effective to all clients. This concern can be allayed by ensuring that, in any design, all clients ultimately receive the treatment hypothesized to be most effective. For example, in waitlist, placebo, or sham designs, clients who first receive one of these treatments instead of the active acupuncture treatment could then be assigned to receive the active acupuncture treatment following the completion of the control treatment. As long as subjects are provided with informed consent that they may first receive a control treatment, and are given information that adequately describes any risks associated with the active or the control treatment, they can decide with full knowledge of the risks and anticipated benefits whether they wish to participate in the clinical trial instead of seeking standard care. It is worth noting that, especially in the case of depression, it is important to select cases for inclusion in the research study that can be ethically subjected to a control treatment. Patients with acute risk (e.g. active suicidal potential in the case of depressed clients) should not be included in clinical trials necessitating a potentially ineffective control condition.

Evaluating Outcome

When evaluating the efficacy of acupuncture in controlled clinical trials, it is essential to remember that Chinese Medicine does not seek to eradicate pathology or fix disorders, but rather to bring the system back into balance. As Schneider & Jonas (1994) have pointed out, treatment outcomes can include at least four categories: *cure* (elimination of disease), *care* (better management of illness), *empowerment* (better sense of ability for self-care and putting illness into context), and *enlightenment* (recognition of one's life purpose as it unfolds). Although acupuncture does focus on both care and cure, it equally values empowerment and enlightenment, two categories that can easily be missed by standard measurement tools. As explained by Paul Houghman: '... (acupuncture) is about helping the whole system adapt with increasing creativity to the environment, so that the individual nature might flourish and feed back its uniqueness into the collective' (Houghman 2000). Appropriate designs for acupuncture clinical trials, as well as other clinical trials, should therefore include measurements of the full spectrum of possible outcomes identified collectively by both conventional and acupuncture practitioners (Bell 2000), in order not to miss 'untargeted' benefits or risks of a treatment (Cella 1992). In addition to standard measures of symptoms such as the Hamilton Rating Scale for Depression (HRSD), it is worth using other measures that tap aspects of how well the participant functions in a variety of domains.

AN ILLUSTRATION OF RESEARCH DESIGN: A PILOT STUDY OF THE EFFICACY OF ACUPUNCTURE IN THE TREATMENT OF MAJOR DEPRESSION

Our pilot study (Allen et al 1998), on which this manual is based, was designed to examine the effectiveness of acupuncture as a treatment for major depression in women. A randomized clinical trial with blind outcome ratings was used to assess women with major depression who were randomly assigned to one of three treatment groups for 8 weeks. *Specific treatment* involved acupuncture treatments for symptoms of depression; *nonspecific treatment* involved acupuncture treatment for symptoms that were not clearly part of the depressive episode; a *waitlist* condition involved waiting without treatment for 8 weeks. Nonspecific and waitlist conditions were followed by crossover to specific treatment.

A community volunteer sample was used, with 33 women who met DSM-IV criteria for current major depressive episode of less than 2 years' duration. Thirty-eight women between the ages of 18 and 45 years were recruited through newspaper advertisements. Advertisements mentioned treatment for depression, but not acupuncture. Participants met criteria for major depression of less than 2 years' duration and did not have other significant psychiatric or medical conditions. Five women (13%) terminated before completion of the study, resulting in a final sample of 33 women who received treatment specifically for depression.[1]

The sample of 33 women had mild-to-moderate depression (mean ±SD 19-item HRSD score 25.1±6.8), with a mean±SD duration of the current episode of 9.2±6.9 months and a history of 2.5±2.9 previous episodes. Additionally, 82% of the participants reported having previously received psychotherapy, 53% reported previous trials of antidepressants, and 11% reported no previous treatment. Some 59% of these participants reported that one or more first-degree relatives also suffered from depression of comparable severity.

Design

As discussed above, factors not specific to acupuncture or the points selected can provide therapeutic impact. Such factors include, among others, the patient–acupuncturist relationship and actively engaging in activity believed to improve depression. The study design therefore provided for the development of two types of acupuncture treatments for each patient: (1) a treatment individually tailored to treat the patient's specific symptoms of depression (specific treatment) and (2) a treatment designed to treat a pattern of disharmony that is not related to the individual's depression, but that is characteristic of the

---

[1]Two terminated for reasons unrelated to treatment (pregnancy and moving out of state), two because of discomfort with the treatment, and one because she was not losing weight and believed that she would lose weight with a pharmacological treatment. This last participant terminated after she had completed nonspecific treatment but before the commencement of specific treatment, and was therefore included in analyses involving the nonspecific treatment. Among these five patients, two terminated from specific treatment, two from nonspecific treatment, and one from waitlist.

individual (nonspecific treatment), such as targeting back pain. The specific and nonspecific treatment were similar from the perspective of the patients, each involving points distributed throughout the same general body regions. Moreover, patients were unaware of which treatment they were receiving. If specific treatments demonstrate greater efficacy than nonspecific treatments, then the effect of acupuncture per se is presumed to be responsible.

The specific and nonspecific treatment plans were developed by an assessing acupuncturist, and were administered by four trained and board-certified acupuncturists other than the assessing acupuncturist. Because the nonspecific treatments involved valid acupuncture points, treating acupuncturists perceived that they were providing a valid treatment, a belief that they would not have held if 'sham' points had been used as a control. The treating acupuncturists were blind to experimental hypotheses and to the nature by which the specific and nonspecific treatments were devised, and were not informed of which treatment plan they received. Nonetheless, it may not be fully appropriate to term this a double-blind study because it remains possible that the acupuncturists may have developed some awareness of the differences between the treatments. On the other hand, the acupuncturists rated their beliefs about the efficacy of the treatment following the first treatment session for each client; these ratings did not differ between specific and nonspecific treatments ($F[1,22] < 1$, ns). Thus, to the extent that we could assess, it appears that this was in fact a double-blind study.

Results

Following treatments specifically designed to address symptoms of depression, 64% of women experienced full remission according to DSM-IV criteria. Comparing the immediate effect of the three 8-week treatment conditions (see Fig. 7.1), patients receiving specific acupuncture treatments demonstrated a significantly ($p < 0.05$) greater reduction in HRSD mean $\pm$ SD scores (-11.7 ± 7.3) than those receiving the nonspecific acupuncture treatments (-2.9 ± 7.9), and showed marginally ($p < 0.12$) greater improvement than waitlist controls (-6.1 ± 10.9). Figure 7.1 summarizes the reduction in depression severity for women in each of the three groups.

Conclusions

Based on a carefully controlled double-blind RCT involving a small outpatient sample of women with major depression, it appears that acupuncture can provide significant symptom relief, at rates

FIGURE 7.1   *Change in depression as a result of acupuncture treatment*

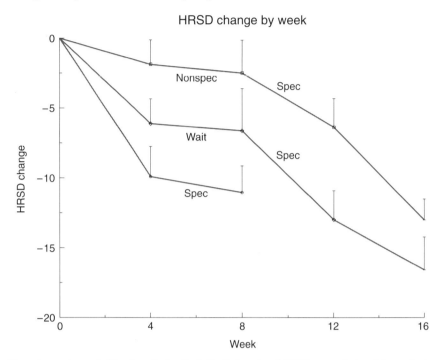

HRSD change by week

Mean ± SEM change in Hamilton Rating Scale for Depression (HRSD) scores for participants in the specific (Spec), nonspecific (NonSpec), and waitlist (Wait) groups by week. Note: After 8 weeks, participants in the NonSpec and Wait groups began receiving specific treatment. After Allen et al (1998), with permission of Blackwell Publishers.

comparable to standard treatments such as psychotherapy or pharmacotherapy. Cross-validation with larger samples and in community clinic settings is required; this treatment manual is designed to facilitate such research.

THE IDEAL PROGRESSION OF RESEARCH

Each of the designs detailed above can have an important role in programmatic research intended to answer the question of whether acupuncture has merit in the treatment of a particular condition. Clinical observation and case studies provide the first evidence that a treatment may be worth researching, and waitlist control studies provide an opportunity to detail those observations more systematically. Controlled trials can then follow that may vary in the degree to which they control all possible confounding factors. Placebo control and sham control trials may control some of the confounding factors, but only a blinded (and we might add a triple-blinded) RCT can provide unequivocal evidence of efficacy. Following positive results in a blinded RCT, trials that examine how acupuncture compares with standard care, or how acupuncture may augment the treatment response when used in addition to standard care, can then provide evidence that assesses how acupuncture may be of use in everyday client care. The advantage of the latter designs is that they may not require blinding. Moreover, if they are conducted *after* efficacy has been established in a tightly controlled trial, they may provide a better estimate of the magnitude of the treatment response in the typical clinical setting.

8 Issues in Implementation

INTRODUCTION

This chapter deals briefly with several issues that will arise in the context of implementing this protocol in research and/or practice. In particular we discuss the handling of acute symptoms that may arise during treatment and the integration of acupuncture with other treatment modalities for cases where clients may be receiving other treatments in addition to acupuncture.

ACUTE SYMPTOMS AND THE DELIVERY OF TREATMENT

When, in the context of working with a specific condition such as depression, an acute situation such as influenza or a cold arises, the practitioner may need to shift the strategy for that specific treatment session. The treatment of deeper imbalances may be contraindicated, especially in the case of active bacterial or viral infections ('external pernicious influences'), without addressing the presenting symptoms. If such an ailment has just begun and the client is not yet doing anything else to address the problem, it is advisable to tailor the treatment to address the presenting situation in the context of the ongoing treatment. It is often possible to modify the treatment while continuing with the main strategy, especially when the patient is already addressing the acute symptoms through other means (e.g. botanical remedies, homeopathy, or medications).

When the 'acute' symptoms are specific to depression – such as increased insomnia or anxiety, changes in appetite, digestive disturbances, or other psychiatric symptoms – the practitioner needs to review the symptoms using the diagnostic framework as outlined in Chapter 5 and modify the treatment to address these changes properly. In the event that the patient is reacting negatively to the initial strategy, care should be taken to assess whether the differentiation of signs and symptoms and the choice of treatment principles accurately match the patient's symptom picture. A reevaluation may be indicated.

Nonpsychiatric Acute Symptoms That May Necessitate a Physician Referral

As in the course of any acupuncture treatment, clients with symptoms that require medical intervention should be promptly referred to a physician. Referral to a physician would be indicated by the presence of any of the following symptoms:

- acute abdominal symptoms

- cardiac conditions

- uncontrolled hypertension

- acute undiagnosed neurological changes

- suspected fracture or dislocation

- acute respiratory distress without previous history.

Clients should be informed before the start of treatment that the acupuncture treatment they will receive is designed to address their symptoms of depression, but that such treatment is not designed to replace the need for a physician should acute medical or psychiatric problems arise.

Acute Psychiatric Symptoms That May Necessitate a Referral

As in the case of acute medical symptoms, the emergence of acute psychiatric symptoms such as psychotic symptoms or suicidal thoughts calls for prompt referral to a mental health specialist.

Psychotic Symptoms

Psychotic symptoms reflect serious problems with reality testing. Psychotic individuals perceive and think about the world in ways that virtually everyone else would consider 'crazy'. Psychotic symptoms most commonly include false beliefs (delusions) and false perceptions (hallucinations). Examples of false beliefs can range from excessive guilt that is delusional (e.g. the belief that the depression is a punishment for sins) to severely delusional beliefs (e.g. aliens are inserting depressive thoughts into the person's head). Hallucinations most often involve hearing voices that others would not hear. Such voices typically say negative things about a depressed person, or provide a negative running commentary on the depressed person's actions.

Mood-congruent psychotic symptoms are delusions or hallucinations of which the content is consistent with typical depressive themes of guilt, inadequacy, death, or deserved punishment. Although many depressed patients report guilt as a symptom, a belief that the depressive illness is punishment for past mistakes is usually characterized as a psychotic feature. It is possible to overlook mood-congruent delusions or hallucinations because they can sometimes be understood in the context of depression; however, when any psychotic symptoms are present, a referral to a licenced mental health professional, such as a psychiatrist or psychologist, is necessary.

Acute Suicidal Symptoms

Clients with depression often have some suicidal thoughts. Although many times these thoughts are fleeting and do not pose a significant danger, the risk of suicide attempt for depressed clients is very real and should be assessed frequently. The practitioner needs routinely to evaluate suicidal thoughts along with other symptoms of depression. This evaluation can be done in a simple, direct, matter-of-fact manner that covers the range of symptoms described below.

Acupuncturists treating depression should become familiar and comfortable with assessing risk of suicide. Moreover, they should become familiar with the state laws that pertain to duty to report and with the limits of clients' confidentiality, and become knowledgeable about referral sources in cases of emergency. It is a good idea to identify a mental health provider that can provide consultation when treating mental health conditions in general, and depression in particular. The risk for depression may be conceptualized in terms of the increasingly serious levels of *thoughts, plan, means,* and *intent* (see Box 8.1).

The assessment of suicide risk progresses along the distinctions shown in Box 8.1. The most natural way to begin inquiry about suicidality is to tie it in with the client's own choice of words describing his or her depression, be it sadness, emptiness, hopelessness, or any other description. The provider can inquire: 'When persons feel [*put the client's descriptors here*], they may think about dying or even killing themselves. Have you?' (Endicott & Spitzer 1978). If the

BOX 8.1	*Assessing the risk of suicide in depressed clients*	
Thoughts	Suicidal thoughts can range from passive thoughts, such as 'I wish I wouldn't wake up', to more active thoughts, such as 'I wish I were dead' or 'The world would be better off if I just killed myself', to even more seriously active thoughts, such as 'I want to kill myself'. Active thoughts typically pose a greater risk than passive thoughts.
Plan	Without a plan on how suicide will be carried out, thoughts alone do not pose an imminent risk (although they may still pose a longer-term risk). The seriousness of the plan can range from a vague plan (e.g. 'Maybe I'd jump off something') to something more concrete (e.g. 'I'd probably jump from a cliff') to the very specific ('I'd asphyxiate myself in the car in the garage'). Greater risk is associated with a more specific plan.
Means	Even if a client has some level of a plan, the risk is realized only if the person has (or can obtain) the means to carry out the plan. If a client indicates a plan (e.g. using a gun), it is important to assess whether the client possesses or could easily obtain the means to carry out the plan (e.g. the practitioner should ask: 'Do you have access to, or plan to get, a gun?'). Having the means to carry out a plan increases the risk.
Intent	Even given a plan and means, some individuals will have no intent to commit suicide, citing reasons such as 'I haven't given up all hope yet' or 'My children need me' or 'My family would be devastated' or 'It's against my religious beliefs'. Intent can be conceptualized in three increasingly risky categories: 1. Intent not to commit suicide 2. Lack of intent not to commit suicide (i.e. some uncertainty) 3. Intent to commit suicide.
Behaviors	Some suicidal behaviors can be preparatory, such as making sure that one's affairs are all in order (e.g. writing a will) or distributing precious belongings to others. These activities may indicate increased risk.

patient's response is quick or defensive, the provider can attempt to put the patient at ease by explaining that these thoughts may come and go. If the client had thoughts of death, the provider's next task is to establish whether these were passive or active thoughts, and to determine whether instruments of suicide are readily available. The third step is to consider whether the patient has ever considered a specific method of suicide and whether or not the client intends to follow through with the suicidal ideas – and why or why not. If the client had considered a specific plan in the past, it is then necessary to inquire about each specific plan, how often it has been considered, and whether the client has ever translated these thoughts into actions, however tentative.

It is also important to keep in mind that some clients' suicidal thoughts and intentions can change rather rapidly. For this reason, all clients should have a list of crisis numbers that they may call. Clients are especially likely to increase their suicidal thoughts and risk if they are under the influence of alcohol. Alcohol, in addition to being a central nervous system depressant, impairs judgement and may increase impulsivity, thereby increasing the risk for suicide. Intoxication by drugs (prescription or illegal) can also increase risk by impairing judgement, by depressing central nervous system function, or (depending on the drug) by serving as a fatal means for attempting suicide. Other important factors that increase the risk are a previous suicide attempt and living alone (or having no one else at home when the suicidal impulses occur). It is important, however, to realize that, even in absence of these risk factors, suicide risk should be taken very seriously. Moreover, even when the client's depressive episode is 'situational', appearing to be an understandable reaction to a serious life condition, the patient is no less likely to die by suicide than a patient in an episode of 'endogenous' etiology (Fawcett et al 1990).

The practitioner is advised to consult with a mental health professional whenever any doubt about the safety of the client arises. Even if a client fails to demonstrate the risk factors listed above, but the practitioner has an intuitive feeling that risk may be present, a consultation is in order. If a client has passive suicidal thoughts and a clear plan not to commit suicide, no consultation is necessary, although it is still encouraged if the practitioner feels that any risk may exist. If more serious thoughts or intent are mentioned, a mental health professional should be contacted immediately – while the client is still in the acupuncturist's office.

The Practitioner–Patient Relationship

In clinical research studies, such as those in which this protocol has been implemented, the practitioner–patient relationship creates unique, and at times difficult, challenges. Central to the concept of randomized control trials (RCTs) is the need to isolate the active components from the nonspecific treatment effects that result from the practitioner–patient relationship. Initially, acupuncture practitioners are skeptical and critical of this attempt, citing that the heart of Chinese Medicine resides in the practitioner's ability to reach the spirit of the patient (Larre & Rochat de la Vallée 1991b). Any clinician knows, through experience and training, that this relationship is at the core of the process of healing, and that it is unrealistic – if not impossible – to assess the clinical effectiveness of a treatment outside of this relationship. There is, however, an invaluable opportunity in research settings to let go of our desire to heal the patient using whatever strategies are available, permitting us to do our best by focusing on the medicine itself, and not on other factors such as the relationship. Within the constraints of a study, when performing an assessment or providing a treatment, we are required to 'stay calm and quiet without special desire' (Larre & Rochat de la Vallée 1991b, p. 16), to do our best, and to let go. It forces us to get out of the way, and to allow the qi to flow naturally on its own, without our expectations mediating the process.

Some implementations of this protocol in research settings may involve a single practitioner conducting assessment and treatment, whereas others (e.g. Allen et al 1998) may involve the use of a separate practitioner for assessment and a separate treatment provider. Assessors and treatment providers must equally be present in themselves when coming in contact with a study participant; precisely because the work of each relies on the work of the other as a team, no one holds an exclusive relationship with the patient. Both have the opportunity to '... let the life of the spirit grow ... and bring this to every part of their work' (Larre & Rochat de la Vallée 1991b, p. 15) without expecting the comfort that this relationship usually affords practitioners in clinical settings; they must therefore rely exclusively on the medicine itself to 'align the will, the purpose, and the spirit of the patient' (Larre & Rochat de la Vallée 1991b). The controlled nature of the treatment provided within a research protocol forces the practitioner to 'needle as if looking into a deep abyss, taking care not to fall' (Su Wen, Ch. 54; cited in Larre & Rochat de la Vallée 1991a), to 'walk on the edge of the mystery of life' with an authentic heart, without fear, and yet cautiously not to fall (Larre & Rochat de la Vallée 1991b, p. 48).

An acupuncturist provides a reference point for the patient to understand his or her signs and symptoms within a bodymind continuum – a framework for validating each person's personal experience of distress or disease. The acupuncturist does not aim to replace the role of a psychotherapist or counselor, but rather strives to become a teacher, an educator, a compass. In the setting of clinical practice, once the initial reframing has been presented and some guidelines for lifestyle and diet modifications have been offered (see Schnyer & Flaws 1998), the acupuncturist hopes to step aside and allow the process of healing to unfold, while continuing to offer his or her presence as guidance and support.

Nevertheless, it is not uncommon (especially when treating psychiatric or emotional conditions) for the patient to attempt to engage the acupuncturist in the role of therapist or counselor. For the acupuncture practitioner, it can be difficult at times not to rely heavily on counseling skills as a way of 'making a signal to reach the spirit of the patient' (Larre & Rochat de la Vallée 1991b, p. 17). Particularly when getting to an impasse in the course of treatment, it is essential for the acupuncturist to delve deeply into the foundations of the medicine in order to reevaluate and further understand the nature of the patient's imbalance. Awakening the will to heal in a patient (Seem 1985) is the key to unfolding the healing process; as expressed by Larre & Rochat de la Vallée (1991b, p. 17): 'Reestablishing the balance always depends on the spirit ... Without the cooperation of the patient inside, you cannot do your work'. The beauty of acupuncture as a treatment, however, resides precisely in its ability to entice the patient's innate potential to heal without the use of words; the language of acupuncture is universal, allowing us to touch the life of a patient even when they cannot talk.

When conducting a controlled treatment study, such as the one for which this manual was originally designed, both assessors and treatment providers were advised to refrain from engaging at a counseling level in any way. All disclosures were viewed as pieces of information that assisted in assessing the nature of the patients' distress, both in terms of their signs and symptoms, and in terms of themselves as unique human beings. Practitioners were asked to refrain from giving advice or suggestions on how to deal with the situation, including dietary and lifestyle changes. In the case of disclosure that suggested suicidal risk, the acupuncturist was advised to follow the guidelines given above. In the research setting, where it is critical to examine the impact of acupuncture per se, and not the participants' reframing of their situation based on discussions with the acupunturist, it is essential that the acupuncturist be warm and present without engaging in reframing or the delivery of advice. In order that participants were able ultimately to benefit from the reframing that is typically part of the acupuncture experience, educational workshops were offered to all study participants after the conclusion of the study, to present the framework and to offer recommendations for maintenance and prevention based on the principles of Chinese Medicine.

ACUPUNCTURE AS AN ADJUNCT TO OTHER TREATMENT MODALITIES

Whereas the efficacy of acupuncture as a treatment for depression is still under study, research has clearly demonstrated that antidepressant medications and specific empirically validated psychotherapies are effective treatments for depression (see Ch. 2). It is therefore ethically indicated that, when a treatment does not result in symptom reduction after an adequate trial, consultation and referrals to mental health specialists are indicated. A good practitioner knows the limit of his or her competence and should be well informed about good consultation and referral sources.

Although a good relationship between the acupuncturist and the patient is very important for the treatment as a whole, psychotherapy and counseling are outside the scope of training and license of most acupuncturists. During the course of acupuncture treatment, some patients might disclose information about difficult issues with which they are dealing. This is a good time gently to suggest adding other treatment modalities, and to provide specific referrals. At present there are no data on the interaction between acupuncture and other treatments for depression. It is not known whether the combination of acupuncture and psychotherapy or acupuncture and antidepressant medications will have a complementary effect that will improve outcome or, conversely, whether the combination treatment will dilute the efficacy of each of its components. It is therefore of utmost importance that treatment providers maintain close communication whenever a patient receives a combination of therapies for depression.

When this manual is used outside a research setting, the acupuncturist is advised, when possible, to work in conjunction with a psychotherapist or counselor. By involving the expertise of a mental healthcare professional, the acupuncturist is allowed to do what acupuncturists do best: engage the qi of the patient. This is not to say that the acupuncturist should avoid developing a therapeutic relationship with the patient that includes, among other skills, an active and caring listening; but rather, it is advised that the acupuncturist should learn to discern when an interdisciplinary effort will better serve the patient. When treating a patient who is also working with a psychotherapist, it may be useful to discuss and coordinate treatment strategies with the therapist. In working with other professionals, it is essential to obtain a written release of information from clients, authorizing the sharing of information between practitioners. Clients have a reasonable expectation of confidentiality (with exceptions in cases of clients posing a danger to self or others), and a release of information is therefore required. Such a release should be signed and dated by the client and should specifically state with whom information may be shared, specifically what information may be shared, and the timeframe covered by the release.

The Treatment Team

In our experience an interdisciplinary effort is best in the care and treatment of people experiencing depression. The treatment team in our studies included acupuncturists, psychotherapists, psychiatrists, and support staff. Study participants were first screened (to determine whether they met inclusion criteria for the study) in a phone interview conducted by psychology students trained specifically for this purpose. People who passed this preliminary screening were assessed by a clinical psychologist who conducted a structured clinical assessment using two widely used instruments, the Structured Clinical Interview for the DSM (SCID) to arrive at the differential diagnosis, and the Hamilton Rating Scale for Depression (HRSD) to obtain a quantitative index of depressive severity. The next step involved a medical screen to rule out medical conditions that may cause depressive symptoms (i.e. hypothyroidism), or unreported or underreported drug use. Following these screenings, participants were assigned to an acupuncture assessor for a Chinese Medicine evaluation, and for the design of an acupuncture treatment plan. The participants were then assigned to an acupuncture treatment provider who performed the treatments in his or her clinical setting. Ongoing monitoring of the care of the participants was then the responsibility of the team comprised of the acupuncture assessor, clinical psychologists, psychology graduate students, and a consulting physician. To assure the quality of assessments, regular supervision meetings took place among all assessors, both acupuncturist and psychologist assessors. Additionally, the core team met regularly to consult about clients, to discuss clinical issues including suicidality, and to make reference to the clinical context.

Future Directions

INTRODUCTION

We have outlined a manualized approach to the treatment of depression, one that is based on the individual's unique experience of depression and that aims to address each particular constellation of signs and symptoms based on pattern differentiation according to Chinese Medicine.

Although the protocol outlined in this manual has been tested in a small sample of women with major depression, much work remains to be done. A larger-scale National Institutes of Health (NIH)-funded clinical trial including men as well as women is currently underway. It has yet to be determined, however, whether acupuncture may be effective in treating chronic or severe depression, or whether it may be useful in treating depression with comorbid disorders such as substance abuse, eating disorders, and anxiety. It is not known whether acupuncture may treat the depressive phase of bipolar disorder, or whether it may be helpful in treating chronic depression or dysthymia.

The long-term prognosis of responders is unknown, and the role of acupuncture as a maintenance treatment needs to be further explored. In acupuncture, after completing a course of treatment, it is generally recommended that people receive maintenance treatments. The frequency and rate of treatments after the acute phase varies, depending on the nature of the condition being treated, the constitutional predisposition of the individual, and their lifestyle choices. As a minimum, acupuncturists would recommend that people receive an acupuncture seasonal 'tune-up' every time the season changes, or approximately four times a year. The concepts of treatment maintenance and continuation are at the core of the practice of Chinese Medicine.

Additionally, it would be worth investigating ways in which acupuncture can assist in facilitating a full recovery from depression. Many individuals who receive treatment for depression are left with a range of residual symptoms. For such people, it would be worth investigating:

- whether the effects of acupuncture alone may be further enhanced by applying it within the context of Chinese Medicine as a complete system – when combined with Chinese herbal medicine and lifestyle and dietary changes

- whether acupuncture may enhance the effect of antidepressants, and whether it may help to counteract some of the adverse side-effects of medications, or reduce the dose of medication required

- whether nonresponders to medication may respond better to acupuncture alone or in combination with medication

- whether combining acupuncture with psychotherapy would enhance the therapeutic effect of either treatment on its own

- whether there may be an enhancement of the therapeutic effect achieved by combining medication, psychotherapy, and acupuncture.

Finally, there are certain populations for which new treatment approaches may be especially welcome. In particular, we will review the need for treatment in three populations for which the use of medication may be difficult: the elderly, women during pregnancy and postpartum, and adolescents.

DEPRESSION IN OLDER ADULTS

Among older adults the prevalence of depression is comparable to that in the general population, but the economic and personal costs may be greater than for younger individuals with depression. Recent community-based (Penninx et al 1998) and primary care clinic-based (Unutzer et al 1997) studies suggest that 10–14% of respondents over age 65 or 70 years suffer from clinically significant depression. Moreover, older individuals with depression incur, on average, almost 50% more healthcare costs in a year's time than do age-matched nondepressed individuals (Unutzer et al 1997), and experience a markedly greater decline in physical capabilities over a 4-year period (Penninx et al 1998). The findings of a recent study suggest that symptoms of depression may function as precursors of future fractures (Whooley et al 1999) as well as diseases diagnosed in the future, and represent a health risk factor comparable in severity to smoking (Shugarman et al 1999). Furthermore, depressive symptomatology may portend cognitive decline in community-dwelling elderly among those with average cognitive function (but not those with high function; Bassuk et al 1998). Finally, suicide rates increase with age and are highest among white men aged 65 years and older (Centers for Disease Control (CDC) 2000a). For every 100 000 people aged 65 years and older, 16.8 committed suicide (Hoyert et al 1999), with men accounting for 83% (CDC 2000a). From 1980 to 1997, the largest relative increases in suicide rates occurred among those aged 80–84 years (CDC 2000a).

For geriatric depression, alternative treatments are additionally important because some traditional interventions may be contraindicated, or not considered acceptable, in the older cohort. Traditional tricyclic antidepressant medications are often not used in the older adults, as they may cause orthostatic hypotension (leading to increased falls and fractures), or because geriatric patients are particularly sensitive to the anticholinergic, cardiovascular, and sedative side effects (NIH Consensus Panel 1992). With respect to newer antidepressant agents, there is a paucity of data on the use of these antidepressants in older patients (Flint 1997). Selective serotonin reuptake inhibitors (SSRIs), which generally produce fewer and more tolerable side effects, are not without problems for use in older adults. SSRIs may induce postural instability in older people, increasing the risk of falls (Laghrissi-Thode et al 1995), and virtually all cases of SSRI-induced hyponatremia have occurred in older people (Liu et al 1996). Whereas in healthy volunteers SSRIs produce no significant cardiac effects, their use in patients with cardiac disease has not been well studied (Sheline et al 1997). Finally, the SSRIs inhibit enzymes involved in the metabolism of a large number of drugs; the result would be that the level of a variety of medications in the blood could be increased when taking these SSRIs (Newhouse 1996), particularly in older adults who, on average, take more medications than their younger counterparts. Acupuncture thus has the potential to offer relief from depression in older adults without the possible risks associated with medication.

DEPRESSION DURING PREGNANCY

Depression is common during pregnancy, with a higher prevalence for depressive symptoms compared with rates of major depressive disorder. Estimated rates for depressive symptoms range between 28% and 34% (O'Hara et al 1984, Rees & Lutkins 1971) with even higher rates (47%) among women of low socioeconomic status (Seguin et al

1995). Despite this documentation of high prevalence, we know relatively little about the onset and course of depression during pregnancy. Kitamura and colleagues (1993) reported onset during pregnancy in about 15% of the depressed pregnant Japanese women they studied. Others (Ballinger 1982, Gotlib et al 1989, 1991) reported that both the incidence and severity of depression during pregnancy increased from the first to the third trimester. Some of these studies also reported that approximately one-third of women who were depressed during pregnancy continued to be depressed after delivery and that half of the women who had postpartum depression were depressed during pregnancy. Moreover, among women who were not clinically depressed during pregnancy, women who became depressed during the postpartum period (4.2%) experienced more depressive symptoms during pregnancy than those who remained nondepressed during the postpartum period (Gotlib et al 1991).

Depression during pregnancy has additional deleterious effects in terms of the wellbeing of the fetus and of the mother following delivery. For example, Orr & Miller (1995) found that among African American women the incidence of preterm delivery was greater in those with more depressive symptoms during pregnancy than in women with few depressive symptoms. Steer and colleagues (1992) reported an increased risk for delivering infants of low birthweight among inner-city women with more depression symptoms compared with those with fewer depression symptoms (20% versus 8%). Similarly they found that, in the same sample, the more depressed women had a greater incidence of preterm delivery (25% versus 8%) and a higher incidence of infants who were smaller than gestational age (15% versus 6%). In terms of the mother's wellbeing, depression during pregnancy is a significant risk factor for postpartum depression (Cutrona 1984, Lum 1990, O'Hara et al 1982, 1984, Pfost et al 1990, Whiffen 1988). Studies in the past two decades have reported that between one-quarter and one-third of women who were depressed during pregnancy experienced depression during the postpartum period as well (Gotlib et al 1989, Watson et al 1984), and maternal postnatal depression has been linked to disturbance in behavior and cognitive development of the infant (Cogill et al 1986, Murray 1992, Whiffen & Gotlib 1989, Wrate et al 1985, Zuckerman & Beardslee 1987). Moreover, maternal depression during the postpartum period can interfere with the normal bonding and attachment process, and compromise the mother's ability to learn effective caretaking and parenting skills (Stein et al 1991, Whiffen & Gotlib 1989, Williams & Carmichael 1985, Wrate et al 1985).

The treatment options available for depressed women during pregnancy are frequently limited. Although psychotherapy is a safe treatment option during pregnancy, it is not readily available in the Health Maintenance Organization (HMO) dominated market and may not be acceptable to all pregnant women. Pharmacological treatments are often not advised during pregnancy; clinical guidelines for the pharmacological treatment of depression during pregnancy recommend that the risks to the woman and fetus associated with no treatment be weighed carefully relative to the risks of treatment (American Psychiatric Association 1993, Coverdale et al 1996, Robert 1996). Physical and behavioral abnormalities have been linked to the use of antidepressant medications during pregnancy (e.g. Ramin et al 1992). Manufacturers of all antidepressants advise that they be avoided during pregnancy, and many women are reluctant to undergo pharmacological treatment for their depression. Consequently depressive symptoms during pregnancy are often tolerated by the patient and remain untreated. Acupuncture holds the potential to offer relief to women experiencing depression during pregnancy without the possible risks associated with medication.

DEPRESSION IN ADOLESCENTS

The incidence of depression in adolescents is close to 20% (Lewinsohn et al 1999). Early onset of depression strongly increases the risk for recurrent depressive disorders during adulthood (Harrington et al 1990, Kovacs 1996, Pine et al 1998, Rao et al 1995), and because depression tends be a chronic and recurrent condition people who experience depression in their teens are likely to experience depression again. Additionally, suicide is the third leading cause of death among people aged 15–24 years (CDC 2000b) and the prevalence of teen suicide is on the increase (CDC 2000a).

A trend towards an earlier age of onset of depression has been observed throughout the twentieth century (Klerman 1990). Major depressive episode is by far the most prevalent affective disorder among adolescents (Lewinsohn et al 1998). Earlier onset of major depression has been associated with being female, with having lower parental education, with the presence of psychiatric comorbidity, and with a history of suicide attempt. In younger children, depression may manifest differently and therefore be missed by conventional diagnostic criteria (Oldenhinkel et al 1999). The rates of adolescent and childhood depression may therefore be seen as conservative estimates (Costello et al 1996, Cooper & Gooyer 1993).

Although suicide attempts among adolescents almost always occur in the context of significant psychopathology (Andrews & Lewinsohn

1992), and the likelihood of suicide attempt increases greatly given the presence of multiple (comorbid) psychiatric disorders (Lewinsohn et al 1998), suicide attempts are still most highly associated with major depression, in conjunction with alcohol and drug use, disruptive behavioral disorders, and anxiety disorders (Lewinsohn et al 1999). Furthermore, the rate of suicide among adolescents is alarmingly high: in 1997 alone 11.4 of every 100,000 adolescents commited suicide and 13.3% of all deaths in this age group are from suicide (Hoyert et al 1999). Moreover, over the 17 years from 1980 to 1997, the rate of suicide increased among all adolescents, but most alarmingly among persons aged 10–14 years, increasing by 109% (CDC 2000a), although the last few years have shown little increase. Based on the Youth Risk Behavior Survey (YRBS) conducted among high-school students by the Centers for Disease Control and Prevention (Kann et al 1998), in 1997 21% of adolescents aged 14–17 years seriously considered suicide and 8% attempted suicide, with 3% of such attempts requiring medical attention; over 1000 young people successfully committed suicide in the United States on that same year. The use of acupuncture in the treatment of depression among adolescents holds the potential not only to address current symptoms, but also to have a significant impact on the developmental trajectory of those who are at a critical juncture in life. Treating depression early in life, at this critical developmental period, is important for several reasons. First, adolescence is a period in which people make important developmental choices, which may be seriously affected by depressive symptoms (Oldenhinkel et al 1999). Second, early onset of depressive disorder strongly increases the risk for recurrent depressive disorder during adulthood (e.g. Harrington et al 1990). Finally, depressive symptoms can lead to unfavorable consequences such as substance abuse and impairment in interpersonal relationships and global functioning (e.g. Birmaher et al 1996).

10 Concluding Remarks

In the course of this book we have attempted to outline an approach for using acupuncture in the treatment of depression, an approach that we hope will find use in clinical practice and research. We have attempted to standardize the approach, in the sense that it can be implemented reliably by any appropriately trained practitioner of acupuncture, but have not standardized it in the sense that all patients would receive the same treatment. Rather, this approach, one of several possible approaches that derive from Chinese Medicine, details how to tailor the treatment to the individual patient. In this respect, we have remained truthful to the fundamental tenets of Chinese Medicine, while also providing a reliable and replicable step-by-step methodology for the implementation of this approach in a variety of clinical and research settings. Many other treatment manuals could be written in a similar vein, for depression as well as for other conditions. The present work provides an example of how to implement acupuncture specifically for any given condition, in a manner that allows for controlled research and for consistency in the clinical setting.

There is much research that remains to be conducted. At this early juncture, it is fair to say that acupuncture offers substantial promise in the treatment of depression. As with many treatments, further research is clearly required to examine the conditions for which acupuncture may be effective. Acupuncture provides yet another choice of treatment for those suffering from depression, and an additional opportunity for those who have failed to respond adequately to other treatments. Furthermore, acupuncture may be especially welcome in cases where treatment with medication is contraindicated, and it may hold promise in enhancing the effects of psychotherapy and pharmacotherapy, while minimizing the unwanted side effects of medications.

In the spirit of finding new possibilities for advancing the treatment of depression and many other illnesses, a comprehensive approach to the art and science of medicine is critically needed, one that draws from diverse therapeutic systems but is also based on solid science. The use of acupuncture in the treatment of depression represents an effort to integrate two very diverse health paradigms; it provides the flexibility needed to address the diverse array of symptoms and experience that plague those with depression, while providing a standardized framework for diagnosis, evaluation, and treatment planning. In the area of research this book represents a stepping-stone towards the development of a new methodology, one that will aim at viewing the patient and the treatment as whole systems, and that will acknowledge the multifactorial and systemic nature of many illnesses, including depression. The development of a manualized approach to acupuncture treatment in clinical trials recognizes the complexity of Chinese Medicine as a system and takes pride on the richness of this tradition.

Clinically, this book hopes to contribute to the area of mental healthcare services by encouraging practitioners of all concerned disciplines '(to) seek the potential within the pathology' (Houghman 2000), to help people move across the healing spectrum from cure to care, to find empowerment and enlightenment in the process of healing, and to reach 'the creative expression of their uniqueness' which is key to survival and health (Houghman 2000). It is hoped that this scientific effort, and this manual in particular, will foster collaboration between psychologists, psychiatrists, and practitioners of Chinese Medicine in their efforts to treat the all too common condition of depression more effectively.

References

Abramson L, Seligman M, Teasdale J 1978 Learned helplessness in humans: critique and reformulation. Journal of Abnormal Psychology 87: 49–74

Allen JJB, Schnyer RN, Hitt SK 1998 The efficacy of acupuncture in the treatment of major depression in women. Psychological Science 9: 397–401

Allen M 1976 Twin studies of affective illness. Archives of General Psychiatry 33: 1475–1478

American Psychiatric Association 1993 Practice guideline for major depressive disorder in adults. American Journal of Psychiatry 150(4): 1–26

American Psychiatric Association 1994 Diagnostic and statistical manual of mental disorders, 4th edn. Washington, DC: APA

Anderson IM, Tomenson BM 1994 The efficacy of selective serotonin re-uptake inhibitors in depression: a meta-analysis of studies against tricyclic antidepressants. Journal of Psychopharmacology 4: 238–249

Andrews JA, Lewinsohn PM 1992 Suicidal attempts among older adolescents: prevalence and co-occurrence with psychiatric disorders. Journal of the American Academy of Child and Adolescent Psychiatry 31: 655–662

Arkowitz H 1992 A common factors therapy for depression. In: Norcross JC, Goldfried MR (eds) Handbook of psychotherapy integration, pp 402–432. New York: Basic Books

Ballinger CB 1982 Emotional disturbance during pregnancy and following delivery. Journal of Psychosomatic Research 26(6): 629–634

Bassuk SS, Berkman LF, Wypij D 1998 Depressive symptomatology and incident cognitive decline in an elderly community sample. Archives of General Psychiatry 55(12): 1073–1081

Beck A 1976 Cognitive therapy and the emotional disorders. New York: International Universities Press

Beekman ATF, Copeland JRM, Prince MJ 1999 Review of community prevalence of depression in later life. British Journal of Psychiatry 174: 307–311

Beinfield H, Korngold E 1991 Between heaven and earth: a guide to Chinese medicine. New York: Ballantine Books

Bell I 2000 Integrative Complementary and Alternative Systems Cancer Research Center grant proposal (1P50Att00436-01). Submitted to the National Institutes of Health for review, March 2000

Belsher G, Costello CG 1988 Relapse after recovery from unipolar depression: a critical review. Psychological Bulletin 104: 84–96

Bensoussan A 1990 Contemporary acupuncture research: the difficulties of research across scientific paradigms. American Journal of Acupuncture 19: 357–365

Berman JS 1980 Social bases of psychotherapy: expectancy, attraction and the outcome of treatment. Dissertation Abstracts International 40: 5800–5801

Birmaher B, Ryan ND, Williamson DE, et al 1996 Childhood and adolescent depression: a review of the past 10 years. Part I. Journal of the American Academy of Child and Adolescent Psychiatry 35: 1427–1439

Blackburn IM, Eunson KM, Bishop S 1986 A two-year naturalistic follow-up of depressed patients treated with cognitive therapy, pharmacotherapy and a combination of both. Journal of Affective Disorders 10: 67–75

Brewington VB, Smith MS, Lipton DL 1994 Acupuncture as a detoxification treatment: an analysis of controlled research. Journal of Substance Abuse Treatment 11: 289–307

Brown GW, Harris TO, Hepworth C 1994 Life events and endogenous depression: a puzzle reexamined. Archives of General Psychiatry 51: 525–534

Brown TA, Barlow DH 1992 Comorbidity among anxiety disorders: implications for treatment and DSM-IV. Journal of Consulting and Clinical Psychology 60: 835–844

Bullock ML, Culliton PD, Olander RT 1989 Controlled trial of acupuncture for severe recidivist alcoholism. Lancet i: 1435–1439

Cassidy CM 1998 Chinese medicine users in the United States. Part I: Utilization, satisfaction, medical plurality. Journal of Alternative and Complementary Medicine 4(1): 17–27

Cella DF 1992 Overcoming difficulties in demonstrating health outcome benefits. Journal of Parenteral and Enteral Nutrition 16: 106–111S

Centers for Disease Control and Prevention 2000a Suicide facts. Online. Available: http://www/cdc/gov/nicpc/factsheets/suifacts.htm 21 August 2000

Centers for Disease Control and Prevention 2000b Suicide. Online. Available http://www/cdc/gov/nicpc/pub-res/FactBok/suicide/htm 21 August 2000

Chang W 1984 Electroacupuncture and ETC. Biological Psychiatry 19: 1271–1272

Chengying Y 1992 Mind-regulating acupuncture treatment of neurosis, using points of Du channel. International Journal of Clinical Acupuncture 3: 193–196

Cherkezova M, Toteva S 1991 Reflexotherapy of patients with associated alcoholism and depressive syndrome. Zhurnal Neuropatologii i Psikhiatrii Imeni SS Korsakova 19(2): 83–84

Cogill S, Capla H, Alexandra H, Robson K 1986 Impact of postnatal depression on the developing child. British Medical Journal 292: 1163–1167

Consensus Conference on Electroconvulsive Therapy 1985 Journal of the American Medical Association 254: 103–108

Cooper PJ, Gooyer I 1993 A community study of depression in adolescent girls I: Estimates of symptom and syndrome prevalence. British Journal of Psychiatry 163: 369–374

Corsini RJ, Wedding D 1989 Current psychotherapies, 4th edn. Itasca: FE Peacock

Costello EJ, Angold A, Burns BJ, et al, 1996 The Great Smokey Mountains Study of Youth: goals, design, methods, and the prevalence of DSM-III-R disorders. Archives of General Psychiatry 53: 1129–1136

Coverdale JH, Chervenak FA, McCullough LB, Bayer T 1996 Ethically justified clinically comprehensive guidelines for the management of the depressed pregnant patient. American Journal of Obstetrics and Gynecology 174: 169–173

Coyne J, Burchill S, Stile SW 1991 An interactional perspective on depression. In: Snyder C, Forsyth F (eds) Handbook of social and clinical psychology, pp 327–349. New York: Pergamon

Cutrona CE 1984 Social support and stress in the transition to parenthood. Journal of Abnormal Psychology 93: 378–390

Denmei S 1990 Introduction to meridian therapy. Seattle: Eastland Press

Delgado PL, Price LH, Heninger GR, Charney DS 1992 Neurochemistry. In: Paykel ES (ed) Handbook of affective disorders, 2nd edn, pp 219–254. New York: Guilford

De-Xin Y 1995 Aging and blood stasis: a new TCM approach to geriatrics. Boulder, Colorado: Blue Poppy Press

Diamond RJ 1998 Instant psychopharmacology: a guide for the non-medical mental health professional. New York: WW Norton

Dobson KS 1989 A meta-analysis of the efficacy of cognitive therapy for depression. Journal of Consulting and Clinical Psychology 57: 414–419

Doogan DP, Caillard V 1992 Sertraline in prevention of depression. British Journal of Psychiatry 160: 217–222

Dunner DL, Dunner PZ 1983 Psychiatry in China: some personal observations. Biological Psychiatry 18: 799–801

Edwards JG 1992 Selective serotonin reuptake inhibitors: a modest though welcome advance in the treatment of depression. British Medical Journal 304: 1644–1646

Edwards JG 1995 Drug choice in depression: selective serotonin reuptake inhibitors or tricyclic antidepressants. CNS Drugs 4: 141–159

Ehlers C, Frank E, Kupfer D 1988 Social zeitgebers and biological rhythms: a unified approach to understanding the etiology of depression. Archives of General Psychiatry 45: 948–952

Eisenberg DM, Kessler RC, Foster C, et al 1993 Unconventional medicine in the United States: prevalence, costs, and patterns of use. New England Journal of Medicine 328: 246–252

Eisenberg DM, Davis RB, Ettner SL, et al 1998 Trends in alternative medicine use in the United States, 1990–1997: results of a follow-up national survey. Journal of the American Medical Association 280(18): 1569–1575

Elkin I, Shea T, Watkins JF, et al 1989 National Institute of Mental Health treatment of depression collaborative program: 1. General effectiveness of treatments. Archives of General Psychiatry 46: 971–982

Endicott J, Spitzer RL 1978 A diagnostic interview: the schedule of affective disorders and schizophrenia. Archives of General Psychiatry 35: 837–844

Evans MD, Hollon SD, DeRubeis RJ, et al 1992 Differential relapse following cognitive therapy and pharmacotherapy for depression. Archives of General Psychiatry 47: 1093–1099

Fawcett J, Scheftner WA, Fogg L, et al 1990 Time-related predictors of suicide in major affective disorder. American Journal of Psychiatry 147(9): 1189–1194

Flaws B 1983 Path of pregnancy. Brookline, Massachusetts: Paradigm

Flaws B 1992 My sister the moon. Boulder, Colorado: Blue Poppy Press

Flaws B 1994 Statements of fact in traditional Chinese medicine. Boulder, Colorado: Blue Poppy Press

Flaws B 1995 The secret of Chinese pulse diagnosis. Boulder, Colorado: Blue Poppy Press

Flaws B 1997 TCM gynecology certification program: supplementary readings. Boulder, Colorado: Blue Poppy Press

Flaws R, Finney D 1996 A compendium of traditional Chinese medicine patterns and treatment. Boulder, Colorado: Blue Poppy Press

Flint AJ 1997 Pharmacologic treatment of depression in late life. Canadian Medical Association Journal 157(8): 1061–1067

Frances A, Manning D, Marin D, Kocsis JH 1992 Relationship of anxiety and depression. Psychopharmacology 106(Suppl): 82–86

Frank E, Kupfer DJ, Perel JM, et al 1990 Three-year outcomes for maintenance therapies in recurrent depression. Archives of General Psychiatry 47(12): 1093–1099

Fruehauf H 1999 Science, politics, and the making of 'TCM': Chinese medicine in crisis. Journal of Chinese Medicine 61: 6–14

Frydrychowski A, Landowski J, Watrobski Z, Ostrowska B 1984 An attempt at applying acupuncture in the treatment of depressive syndromes. Psychiatria Polska 18: 247–250

Glen AI 1984 Continuation therapy with lithium and amitriptyline in unipolar depressive illness: a randomized, double-blind, controlled trial. Psychological Medicine 41: 37–50

Goodwin GM 1992 Tricyclic and newer antidepressants. In: Paykel ES (ed) Handbook of affective disorders, 2nd edn, pp 327–344. New York: Guilford

Gotlib IH, Beach SR 1995 A marital/family discord model of depression. In: Jacobson NS, Gurman AS (eds) Clinical handbook of couple therapy, pp 411–436. New York: Guilford

Gotlib IH, Whiffen VE, Mount JH, Milne K, Cordy NI 1989 Prevalance rates and demographic characteristics associated with depression during pregnancy and the postpartum. Journal of Consulting and Clinical Psychology 57: 269–274

Gotlib IH, Whiffen VE, Mount JH 1991 Prospective investigation of postpartum depression: factors involved in onset and recovery. Journal of Abnormal Psychology 100: 122–132

Greenberg R, Fisher S 1997 Mood-mending medicines: probing drug, psychotherapy, and placebo solutions. In: Fisher S, Greenberg R (eds) From placebo to panacea: putting psychiatric drugs to the test, pp 57–97. New York: John Wiley

Greenberg RP, Bornstein RF, Greenberg MD, Fisher S 1992 A meta-analysis of anti-depressant outcome under 'blinder' conditions. Journal of Consulting and Clinical Psychology 60: 664–669

Greenberg RP, Bornstein RF, Zborowski MJ, Fisher S, Greenberg MD 1994 A meta-analysis of fluoxetine outcome in the treatment of depression. Journal of Nervous and Mental Disease 182: 547–551

Grencavage L, Bootzin R, Shoham V 1993 Specific and nonspecific effects of therapy. In: Costello CG (ed) Basic issues in psychopathology, pp 359–376. New York: Wiley

Hamilton M 1967 Development of a rating scale for primary depressive illness. British Journal of Social Psychology 6: 278–296

Hammen C 1991 The generation of stress in the course of unipolar depression. Journal of Abnormal Psychology 100: 555–561

Hammer L 1990 Dragon rises, red bird flies: psychology and Chinese medicine. New York: Station Hill Press

Hammerschlag R 1998 Methodological and ethical issues in clinical trials of acupuncture. Journal of Alternative and Complementary Medicine 4: 159–171

Han JS 1986 Electroacupuncture: an alternative to antidepressants for treating affective diseases? International Journal of Neuroscience 29: 79–92

Harrington R, Fudge H, Rutter M, Pickles A, Hill J 1990 Adult outcomes of childhood and adolescent depression. I. Psychiatric status. Archives of General Psychiatry 47: 465–473

Hiller W, Zaudig M, von Bose M 1989 The overlap between depression and anxiety on different levels of psychopathology. Journal of Affective Disorders 16: 223–231

Hirschfeld RMA, Schatzberg AF 1994 Long-term management of depression. American Journal of Medicine 97(Suppl 6A): 33S–38S

Hollon S, Garber J 1988 Cognitive therapy. In: Social cognition and clinical psychology. New York: Guilford

Hougham P 2000 More than skin deep – acupuncture in mental health. The Matthew Trust Holistic Care Conference for the Mentally Ill, 12 May 2000, House of Lords, York, UK

Hoyert DL, Kochanek KD, Murphy SL 1999 Deaths: final data for 1997. National Vital Statistics Report, 47(19). DHHS publication no. (PHS) 99–1120. Hyattsville, Maryland: National Center for Health Statistics

Jarrett LS 1999 The inner tradition of Chinese Medicine. Stockbridge: Spirit Path Press

Kann K, Kinchen S, Williams BI, et al 1998 Youth risk behavior surveillance – United States, 1997. CDC Mortality and Morbidity Weekly Report 47(SS-3), 1–89. Online. Available: http://cdc.gov/MMWR/htm

Kaptchuk TJ 1983 The web that has no weaver: understanding Chinese medicine. New York: Congdon & Weed

Kaptchuk TJ 1987 Jade Pharmacy clinical manual. California: Ming-men Designs

Kaptchuk TJ 1989 Lectures notes. Stanford, Connecticut: Tri-State Institute of Traditional Chinese Acupuncture

Kaptchuk TJ 2000 The web that has no weaver: understanding Chinese Medicine, 2nd edn. Chicago: Contemporary Books

Kasper S, Fuger J, Moller HJ 1992 Comparative efficacy of antidepressants. Drugs 43: 11–23

Keltner NL, Folks DG 1997 Psychotropic drugs, 2nd edn. St Louis, Missouri: Mosby-Year Book

Kessler RC, McGonagle KA, Shanyang Z, et al 1994 Lifetime and 12-month prevalence of DSM-III-R psychiatric disorders in the United States: results from the National Comorbidity Study. Archives of General Psychiatry 51: 8–19

Kirsch I, Sapirstein G 1998 Listening to Prozac but hearing placebo: a meta-analysis of antidepressant medication. Prevention and Treatment 1, June 26. Online. Available: http://journals.apa.org/.prevention

Kitamura T, Shima SS, Sugawara M, et al 1993 Psychological and social correlates of the onset of affective disorders among pregnant women. Psychological Medicine 23: 967–975

Klerman GL 1990 The current age of youthful melancholia: evidence of increase in depression among adolescents and young adults. British Journal of Psychiatry 152: 4–14

Klerman GL, Dimascio A, Weissman M 1974 Treatment of depression by drugs and psychotherapy. American Journal of Psychiatry 131: 186–191

Kovacs M 1996 Presentation and course of major depresive disorder during childhood and later years of the life span. Journal of the American Academy of Child and Adolescent Psychiatry 35: 705–715

Laghrissi-Thode F, Pollock BG, Miller M, Altieri L, Kupfer DJ 1995 Comparative effects of sertraline and nortriptyline on body sway in older depressed patients. American Journal of Geriatric Psychiatry 3: 217–228

Lambert MJ, Bergin AE 1994 The effectiveness of psychotherapy. In: Bergin AE, Garfield SL (eds) Handbook of psychotherapy and behavior change, 4th edn, pp 143–189. New York: Wiley

Larre C, Rochat de la Vallée E 1985 The secret treatise of the spiritual orchid. London: British Register of Oriental Medicine

Larre C, Rochat de la Vallée E 1991a The heart in lingshu, Chapter 8. Cambridge, Massachusetts: Monkey Press

Larre C, Rochat de la Vallée E 1991 The practitioner–patient relationship. Journal of Traditional Acupuncture 14–17: 48–50

Larre C, Rochat de la Vallée E 1995 Rooted in spirit: the heart of Chinese medicine. New York: Station Hill Press

Larre C, Rochat de la Vallée E 1996 The seven emotions: psychology and health in ancient China. Cambridge, Massachusetts: Monkey Press

Larsen J 1991 MAOIs in the treatment of depression: a review. European Journal of Psychiatry 5: 79–88

Lewinsohn PM, Hoberman H, Teri L, Hautzinger M 1985 An integrative theory of depression. In: Reiss S, Bootzin R (eds) Theoretical issues in behavior therapy, pp 264–284. New York: Academic Press

Lewinsohn PM, Rohde P, Seeley JR 1998 Major depressive disorders in older adolescents: prevalence, risk factors, and clinical implications. Clinical Psychology Review 18: 765–794

Lewinsohn PM, Rohde P, Klein DN, Seeley JR 1999 Natural course of adolescent major depressive disorder: I. Continuity into young adulthood. Journal of the American Academy of Child and Adolescent Psychiatry 38(1): 56–63

Liu BA, Mittmann N, Knowles SR, Shear NH 1996 Hyponatremia and the syndrome of inappropriate secretion of antidiuretic hormone associated with the use of selective serotonin reuptake inhibitors: a review of spontaneous reports. Canadian Medical Association Journal 155: 519–527

Low R 1983 The extraordinary vessels of accupuncture: an account of their energies, meridians and control points. Wellingsborough, UK: Thorson

Lum CU 1990 A relationship of demographic variables, antepartum depression, and stress to postpartum depression. Journal of Clinical Psychology 46: 588–592

Maciocia G 1987 Tongue diagnosis in Chinese medicine. Seattle: Eastland Press

Maciocia G 1989 The foundations of Chinese medicine. London: Churchill Livingstone

Maciocia G 1994 The practice of Chinese medicine: the treatment of diseases with acupuncture and Chinese herbs. London: Churchill Livingstone

McLellan AT, Grossman DS, Blaine JD, Haverkos HW 1993 Acupuncture treatment for drug abuse: a technical review. Journal of Substance Abuse Treatment 10: 569–576

Mann F 1973 Acupuncture, the ancient Chinese art of healing and how it works scientifically, 2nd edn. New York: Vintage Books

Mannuzza S, Fyer AJ, Martin LY, et al 1989 Reliability of anxiety assessment. Archives of General Psychiatry 46: 1093–1101

Matsumoto K, Birch S 1988 Hara diagnosis: reflections on the sea. Brookline, Massachusetts: Paradigm

Maxmen JS, Ward NG 1995 Psychotropic drugs: fast facts. New York: WW Norton

Mendlewicz J, Ranier J 1977 Adoption study supporting genetic transmission in manic-depressive illness. Nature 168: 327–329

Merikangas KR, Gelernter CS 1990 Comorbidity for alcoholism and depression. Psychiatric Clinics of North America 12: 613–632

Montgomery SA, Dufour H, Brion S, et al 1988 The prophylactic efficacy of fluoxetine in unipolar depression. British Journal of Psychiatry 153(Suppl 3): 69–73

Murphy JM, Monson RR, Olivier DC, et al 1987 Affective disorders and mortality. Archives of General Psychiatry 44: 473–480

Murray L 1992 The impact of postnatal depression on infant development. Journal of Child Psychology and Psychiatry 33: 543–561

Murry CJL, Lopez AD 1996 The global burden of disease. Boston, Massachusetts: Harvard School of Public Health

Newhouse PA 1996 Use of serotonin selective reuptake inhibitors in geriatric depression. Journal of Clinical Psychiatry 57a(Suppl 5): 12–22

Newmeyer JA, Johnson G, Klot S 1984 Acupuncture as a detoxification modality. Journal of Psychoactive Drugs 16: 241–261

NIH Consensus Development Panel on Depression in Late Life 1992 Journal of the American Medical Association 268: 1018–1024

Nolen-Hoeksema S 1987 Sex differences in unipolar depression: evidence and theory. Psychological Bulletin 101: 259–282

O'Connor J, Bensky D, trans. 1981 Acupuncture: a comprehensive text. Shanghai College of Traditional Chinese Medicine. Seattle: Eastland Press

O'Hara MW, Rehm LP, Campbell SB 1982 Predicting depressive symptomatology; cognitive behavioral models and postpartum depression. Journal of Abnormal Psychology 91: 457–461

O'Hara MW, Neunaver DJ, Zekoski EM 1984 Prospective study of postpartum depression: prevalance, course, and predictive factors. Journal of Abnormal Psychology 93: 158–171

Oldenhinkel AJ, Wittchen HU, Schuster P 1999 Prevalence, 20-month incidence and outcome of unipolar depressive disorders in a community sample of adolescents. Psychological Medicine 29: 655–668

Oleson TD 1992 Auriculotherapy manual: Chinese and Western systems of ear acupuncture. Los Angeles, California: Health Care Alternatives

Oltmans TF, Emery RE 1995 Abnormal psychology. Upper Saddle River: Prentice Hall

Orr ST, Miller CG 1995 Maternal depressive symptoms and the risk of poor pregnancy outcome: review of the literature and preliminary findings. Epidemiological Reviews 17(1): 165–171

Pine DS, Cohen P, Gurley D, Brook J, Ma Y 1998 The risk for early-adulthood anxiety and depressive disorders in adolescents with anxiety and depressive disorders. Archives of General Psychiatry 55: 56–64

Penninx BWJH, Guralnik JM, Ferrucci L, et al 1998 Depressive symptoms and physical decline in community-dwelling older persons. Journal of the American Medical Association 279: 1720–1726

Petrie JP, Hazleman BL 1986 A controlled study of acupuncture in neck pain. Journal of Rheumatology 25: 271–275

Pfost KS, Stevens MJ, Lum CU 1990 The relationship of demographic variables, antepartum depression, and stress to postpartum depression. Journal of Clinical Psychology 46(5): 588–592

Polyakov SE 1987 Acupuncture in the treatment of endogenous depression. Zhurnal Nevropatologii i Psikhiatrii Imeni SS Korsakova 87: 604–608

Polyakov SE 1988 Acupuncture in the treatment of endogenous depressions. Soviet Neurology and Psychiatry 21: 36–44

Polyakov SE, Dudaeva KI 1990 Neurophysiological changes in reflex therapy for endogenous depression. Zhurnal Nevropatologii i Psikhiatrii Imeni SS Korsakova 90: 99–103

Porkert M 1983 The essentials of Chinese diagnosis. Zurich: Chinese Medicine Publications

Prange AJ, Wilson IC, Lynn CW, Lacoe BA, Stikeleather RA 1974 L-Tryptophan in mania – contribution to a permissive hypothesis of affective disorders. Archives of General Psychiatry 30: 56–62

Prien RF, Kupfer DJ 1986 Continuation drug therapy for major depression episodes: how long should it be maintained? American Journal of Psychiatry 143: 18–23

Prien RF, Kupfer DJ 1984 Drug therapy in the prevention of recurrences in unipolar and bipolar affective disorders: a report of the NIMH Collaborative Study Group comparing lithium carbonate, imipramine, and a lithium carbonate–imipramine combination. Archives of General Psychiatry 41: 1096–1104

Ramin SM, Bertis B, Little MA, Gilstrap LCI 1992 Psychotropics in pregnancy. In: Gilstrap LC, Little BB (eds) Drugs and pregnancy, pp 145–173. New York: Elsevier Science

Rao U, Ryan ND, Birmaher B, et al 1995 Unipolar depression in adolescents: clinical outcome in adulthood. Journal of the American Academy of Child and Adolescent Psychiatry 34: 566–578

Requena Y 1986 Terrains and pathology in acupuncture, vol. 1. Brookline, Massachusetts: Paradigm

Rees WD, Lutkins SD 1971 Parental depression before and after childbirth. Journal of the Royal College of General Practitioners 21: 20–31

Robert E 1996 Treating depression in pregnancy. New England Journal of Medicine 335: 1056–1058

Robinson DS, Lerfald SC, Bennett B, et al 1991 Continuation and maintenance treatment of major depression with the monoamineoxidase inhibitor phenelzine: a double-blind placebo-controlled discontinuation study. Psychopharmacological Bulletin 27: 31–39

Robinson LA, Berman JS, Neimeyer RA 1990 Psychotherapy for the treatment of depression: a comprehensive review of controlled outcome research. Psychological Bulletin 100: 30–49

Rush AJ, Weissenburger JE 1994 Melancholic symptom features and DSM-IV. American Journal of Psychiatry 151: 489–498

Sackheim HA 1989 Mechanisms of action. Convulsive Therapy 6: 207–310

Schneider CJ, Jonas WB 1994 Are alternative treatments effective? Issues and methods involved in measuring effectiveness of alternative treatments. Subtle Energies 5: 69–92

Schnyer RN, Allen JJB 2001 Depression and mental illness. In: Cassidy CM, Micozzi M (eds) Contemporary practice of acupuncture and oriental medicine. WB Saunders

Schnyer R, Flaws B 1998 Curing depression naturally with Chinese medicine. Boulder, Colorado: Blue Poppy Press

Seem M 1985 Lectures notes. Stanford, Connecticut: Tri-State Institute of Traditional Chinese Acupuncture

Seem M 1987 Bodymind energetics: towards a dynamic model of health. Rochester, Vermont: Thorson

Seem M 1990 Acupuncture imaging: perceiving the energetic pathways of the body. Rochester, Vermont: Healing Arts Press

Seem M 1993 A new American acupuncture: acupuncture osteopathy. Boulder, Colorado: Blue Poppy Press

Seguin L, Potvin I, St Denis M, Loiselle J 1995 Chronic stressors, social support, and depression during pregnancy. Obstetrics and Gynecology 85: 583–589

Seligman M 1975 Helplessness: on depression, development, and death. San Francisco, California: Freeman

Seligman M, Nolen-Hoeksema S 1987 Explanatory style and depression. In: Psychopathology: an interactional perspective, pp 125–139. New York: Academic Press

Shea T, Elkin I, Imber SD, et al 1992 Course of depressive symptoms over follow-up: findings from the National Institute of Mental Health Treatment of Depression Collaborative Research Program. Archives of General Psychiatry 49: 782–787

Sheline YI, Freedland KE, Carney RM 1997 How safe are serotonin reuptake inhibitors for depression inpatients with coronary heart disease? American Journal of Medicine 102: 54–59

Shelton R, Hollon S, Purdon S, Loosen P 1991 Biological and psychological aspects of depression. Behavior Therapy 22: 201–228

Shugarman L, Buttar A, Blaum C, Fries B 1999 Risk factors associated with hospitalization in a home and community-based population. Paper presented to the 1999 annual meeting of the Gerontological Society of America, November, San Francisco, California, 19–23 November 1999

Siever L, Davis K 1985 Overview: toward a dysregulation hypothesis of depression. American Journal of Psychiatry 142: 1017–1028

Spitzer RL, Williams JBW, Gibbon M, First MB 1990 Structured clinical interview for DSMIIIR (SCID). Washington, DC: American Psychiatric Press

Steer RA, Scholl TO, Hediger ML, Fischer RL 1992 Self-reported depression and negative pregnancy outcomes. Journal of Clinical Epidemiology 45: 1093–1099

Stein A, Gath DH, Bucher J, et al 1991 The relationship between postnatal depression and mother–child interaction. British Journal of Psychiatry 158: 46–52

Steinbrueck SM, Maxwell SE, Howard GS 1983 A meta-analysis of psychotherapy and drug therapy in the treatment of unipolar depression with adults. Journal of Consulting and Clinical Psychology 51: 856–863

Stoll AL, Severus WE, Freeman MP, et al 1999 Omega 3 fatty acids in bipolar disorder: a preliminary double-blind, placebo-controlled trial. Archives of General Psychiatry 56: 407–412

Streitberger K, Kleinhenz J 1998 Introducing a placebo needle into acupuncture research. Lancet 352: 364–365

Strober M, Morrell W, Burroughs J, et al 1988 A family study of bipolar I disorder in adolescence: early onset of symptoms linked to increased familial loading and lithium resistance. Journal of Affective Disorders 15: 255–268

Suobin K 1991 Clinical observation on 103 cases of neurasthenia treated with plum-blossom needle tapping. International Journal of Clinical Acupuncture 2: 419–421

Thase ME 1990 Relapse and recurrence in unipolar major depression: short-term and long-term approaches. Journal of Clinical Psychiatry 51: 51–57; discussion 58–59

Toteva S 1991 Reflexotherapy of patients with associated alcoholism and depressive syndrome. Zhurnal Neuropatologii i Psikhiatrii Imeni SS Korsakova 19: 83–84

Ulett GA 1992 3000 years of acupuncture: from metaphysics to neurophysiology. Integrative Psychiatry 8: 91–100

Unutzer J, Patrick DL, Simon G, et al 1997 Depressive symptoms and the cost of health services in HMO patients aged 65 years and older. Journal of the American Medical Association 277: 1618–1623

Watson JP, Elliot SA, Rugg AJ, Brough DI 1984 Psychiatric disorder in pregnancy and the first postnatal year. British Journal of Psychiatry 144: 453–462

Wender PH, Kety SS, Rosenthal D, et al 1986 Psychiatric disorders in the biological and adoptive families of individuals with affective disorders. Archives of General Psychiatry 43: 923–929

Whooley MA, Kip KE, Cauley JA, et al 1999 Depression, falls, and risk of fracture in older women. Archives of Internal Medicine 159: 484–490

Whiffen VE 1988 Vulnerability to postpartum depression: a prospective multivariate study. Journal of Abnormal Psychology 97: 467–474

Whiffen VE, Gotlib IH 1989 Infants of postpartum depressed mothers: temperament and cognitive status. Journal of Abnormal Psychology 98: 274–279

Whybrow P, Akiskal H, McKinney W 1984 Mood disorders: toward a new psychobiology. New York: Plenum

Williams H, Carmichael A 1985 Depression in mothers in a multi-ethnic urban industrial municipality in Melbourne: aetiological factors and effects on infants and pre-school children. Journal of Child Psychology and Psychiatry 26: 277–288

Wiseman N, Feng Y 1998 A practical dictionary of Chinese medicine, 2nd edn. Brookline, Massachusetts: Paradigm

Wolfe H 1998 Managing menopause naturally with Chinese medicine. Boulder, Colorado: Blue Poppy Press

World Health Organization 1992 ICD-10 classification of mental and behavioural disorders: clinical descriptions and diagnostic guidelines. Geneva: WHO

Wrate RM, Roonew AC, Thomas PF, Cox JL 1985 Postnatal depression and child development: a three-year follow up study. British Journal of Psychiatry 146: 622–627

Xinnong C (ed) 1987 Chinese acupuncture and moxibustion. Beijing: Foreign Language Press

Zimmerman M, Pfohl B, Coryell WH, Corenthal C, Stangl D 1991 Major depression and personality disorder. Journal of Affective Disorders 22: 199–210

Zuckerman BS, Beardslee WR 1987 Maternal depression: a concern for pediatricians. Pediatrics 79: 110–117

Appendix A

Intake Form

Please help us provide you with a complete evaluation by taking the time to fill out this questionnaire carefully. If there is anything you wish to bring to our attention which is not asked on this form, please note it in the comment section. Thank you.

Name: .... Age: ....

Address: ....

.... Zip: ....

Phone: (home) .... (work) ....

Place of Birth: .... Occupation: ....

Marital Status: Single   Married   Divorced   Partnership   Children/Ages ....

Height: .... Weight: .... Blood Pressure: ....

Today's Date: ....

What is the **main problem** that brings you here today?

Assessor's Notes:

How long ago did this problem begin and what precipitated it? (be specific)

Assessor's Notes:

In what way and to what extent does this problem affect your daily activities?

Assessor's Notes:

What would happen if your condition would change? In what way would you be different?

Assessor's Notes:

Other related or apparently unrelated difficulties or problems:

Assessor's Notes:

What areas do you feel tend to become vulnerable when tired or under stress?

Assessor's Notes:

Past medical history (significant illnesses for which you have received medication, surgery, hospitalization. Please include date.)

Assessor's Notes:

Significant trauma (accidents, falls, etc.)

Assessor's Notes:

Allergies (seasonal, drugs, chemicals, food, etc.)

Assessor's Notes:

Birth history – your own (prolonged labor, premature birth, etc.)

Assessor's Notes:

Family medical history (parents, grandparents, siblings)

Assessor's Notes:

Any serious or communicable conditions (HIV, hepatitis, epilepsy)

Assessor's Notes:

Are you presently under the care of a physician?
Physician's name

Assessor's Notes:

Are you presently on medication?
If so, what?

Assessor's Notes:

Vitamins, herbs, nutritional supplements, other:

Assessor's Notes:

Do you exercise? Please describe:

Assessor's Notes:

Coffee, alcohol, recreational drugs, tobacco; how often and how much?

Assessor's Notes:

Comments:

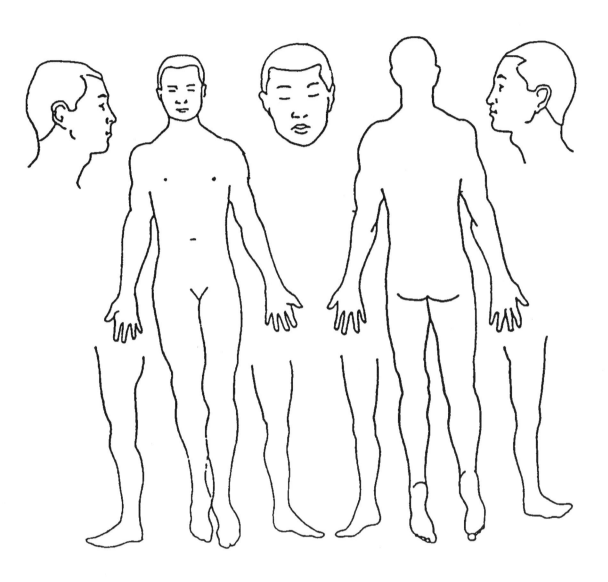

Intake form for the research project *Acupuncture in the Treatment of Depression*   ©1999–2000, Rosa N. Schnyer

Please indicate which symptoms you have experienced DURING THE LAST 2 WEEKS. In the lines where there are two or more options circle those applicable; for example: *moodiness/mood swings/feelings of frustration*.
Rate them according to their severity and frequency.
DO RATE ALL ITEMS THAT ARE APPLICABLE TO YOU.
In addition, for women, mark on the left with an asterisk (*) the symptoms that worsen around the time of your period.

0	**absent**
1	**mild (infrequent or not intense)**
2	**moderate (frequent or more intense)**
3	**severe (constant or very intense)**

For Client to Complete

Last 2 weeks!

	Absent	Mild	Moderate	Severe	For acupuncturist to complete
LvQiStag					
___ moodiness/mood swings/feelings of frustration	0	1	2	3	
___ snapping easily/feeling wound up	0	1	2	3	
___ colds hands/feet (that warm up when relaxed)	0	1	2	3	
___ sensation of a lump in the throat	0	1	2	3	
___ pains that are vague or change location	0	1	2	3	
___ muscle cramps, twitches, spasms	0	1	2	3	
___ tension in neck, jaw, shoulders, hips	0	1	2	3	
___ distension or fullness in the abdomen, breast, rib cage	0	1	2	3	
___ discomfort or pain in the stomach and epigastrium	0	1	2	3	
___ nausea	0	1	2	3	
___ hiccups, belching, burping, flatulence	0	1	2	3	Total Score
___ gas pains, tension in stomach/intestines	0	1	2	3	of LvQiStag
___ irritability	0	1	2	3	symptoms ....
LvQiStag–Ht/Lu					
___ chest oppression/fullness	0	1	2	3	
___ frequent sighing/breathlessness	0	1	2	3	Total Score
___ tearful, weepy	0	1	2	3	of LvQiStag–Ht/Lu
___ easily affected by others' problems	0	1	2	3	symptoms ....
LvQiStag–Heat					
___ irritability with agitation/sensation of heat in the chest	0	1	2	3	
___ mental restlessness	0	1	2	3	
___ irascibility/explosiveness/easy anger	0	1	2	3	Total Score
___ aggression/violent outbursts of anger	0	1	2	3	of LvQiStag–Heat
___ bitter taste in the mouth	0	1	2	3	symptoms ....

Intake form for the research project *Acupuncture in the Treatment of Depression*   ©1999–2000, Rosa N. Schnyer

For Client to Complete					
Last 2 weeks!					

	Absent	Mild	Moderate	Severe	For acupuncturist to complete
Shendist					
__ insomnia:					
__ with difficulty falling asleep	0	1	2	3	
__ with difficulty staying asleep	0	1	2	3	
__ with restless sleep	0	1	2	3	
__ vivid, excessive or disturbing dreams	0	1	2	3	
__ excessive desire to sleep	0	1	2	3	
__ palpitations	0	1	2	3	
__ anxiety	0	1	2	3	
__ poor memory	0	1	2	3	
__ easily startled or frightened	0	1	2	3	
__ easily confused or disoriented	0	1	2	3	
__ trouble finding the right words	0	1	2	3	
__ dullness of thought	0	1	2	3	
__ easily moved to tears or laughter	0	1	2	3	Total Score of Shendist
__ heart palpitations prompted or worsened by fatigue or exercise	0	1	2	3	symptoms ....
Qivac–Sp					
__ weakness/lethargy/fatigue	0	1	2	3	
__ poor appetite	0	1	2	3	
__ weak digestion	0	1	2	3	
__ lack of strength in the extremities	0	1	2	3	
__ tendency towards loose stools or diarrhea	0	1	2	3	Total Score
__ abdominal distension	0	1	2	3	of Qivac–Sp
__ fatigue after eating	0	1	2	3	symptoms ....
Yangvac–Sp					
__ chilled extremities (that don't warm up when relaxed)	0	1	2	3	
__ feeling frequently cold	0	1	2	3	Total Score
__ lack of motivation	0	1	2	3	of Yangvac–Sp
__ excessive desire to sleep	0	1	2	3	symptoms ....

Intake form for the research project *Acupuncture in the Treatment of Depression*   ©1999–2000, Rosa N. Schnyer

For Client to Complete

Last 2 weeks!

	Absent	Mild	Moderate	Severe	For acupuncturist to complete
Qivac–Lu					
__ shortness of breath	0	1	2	3	
__ spontaneous perspiration	0	1	2	3	Total Score
__ cough upon exertion or talking	0	1	2	3	of Qivac–Lu
__ no desire to talk	0	1	2	3	symptoms ....
Qivac–Kd					
__ low back soreness	0	1	2	3	
__ knee soreness	0	1	2	3	
__ frequent urination	0	1	2	3	
__ night urination	0	1	2	3	
__ low sexual interest	0	1	2	3	Total Score
__ loss of hair	0	1	2	3	of Qivac–Kd
__ pronounced sensitivity to cold	0	1	2	3	symptoms ....
Yinrepletion–Dampness					
__ edema/water retention	0	1	2	3	
__ puffy eyes/face/ankles/hands	0	1	2	3	
__ feelings of heaviness in the head/abdomen/limbs	0	1	2	3	
__ sore muscles	0	1	2	3	
__ fullness of the head with mucus	0	1	2	3	
__ no desire to drink liquids	0	1	2	3	
__ excessive mucus in the back of the throat/postnasal drip	0	1	2	3	
__ frequent mucous congestion in nose or throat	0	1	2	3	
__ cloudy, copious urination	0	1	2	3	
__ diarrhea	0	1	2	3	
__ copious vaginal discharge	0	1	2	3	
__ sticky discharges from eyes, ears, nose, throat	0	1	2	3	
__ skin eruptions filled with fluid	0	1	2	3	
__ feel worse in humid environment or from eating greasy, fatty foods, milk products, sugar, eggs	0	1	2	3	Total Score of Yinrepletion–
__ dullness of thought with a fuzzy head	0	1	2	3	Dampness
__ tendency towards obsessive thinking or rumination	0	1	2	3	symptoms ....
Bloodvac–Lv					
__ numbness of the limbs	0	1	2	3	Total Score
__ blurred vision	0	1	2	3	of Bloodvac–Lv
__ difficulty seeing at night	0	1	2	3	symptoms ....

Intake form for the research project *Acupuncture in the Treatment of Depression*   ©1999–2000, Rosa N. Schnyer

For Client to Complete

Last 2 weeks!

	Absent	Mild	Moderate	Severe	For acupuncturist to complete
Yinvac					
__ feeling flushed, specially in the afternoon	0	1	2	3	
__ heat in the palms, the soles, the chest	0	1	2	3	
__ night sweats	0	1	2	3	
__ symptoms worst in the evening	0	1	2	3	
__ hot flushes	0	1	2	3	
__ scanty urination	0	1	2	3	
__ sore throat when fatigued or overtired	0	1	2	3	
__ dry mucous membranes, skin, eyes, hair	0	1	2	3	Total Score
__ lack of sexual secretions (women)	0	1	2	3	of Yinvac
__ spontaneous sexual emissions (men)	0	1	2	3	symptoms ....
Vacuityheat					
__ any of the symptoms in the above group, but very severe	0	1	2	3	Total Score
__ in addition to symptoms above, aggressive and impatient	0	1	2	3	of Vacuityheat
__ hypersensitive	0	1	2	3	symptoms ....
Yangrepletion					
__ excessive thirst	0	1	2	3	
__ excessive hunger	0	1	2	3	
__ constipation	0	1	2	3	
__ bleeding gums	0	1	2	3	
__ sores in the mouth or tongue	0	1	2	3	
__ throbbing splitting headaches	0	1	2	3	
__ severe dizziness, vertigo, ringing in the ears	0	1	2	3	
__ genital swelling or itching	0	1	2	3	Total Score
__ abnormal, excessive vaginal discharge	0	1	2	3	of Yangrepletion
__ restlessness accompanied by compulsive behavior	0	1	2	3	symptoms ....
AdditsymptLv					
__ pain in the diaphragm, ribs, groin, pelvic region	0	1	2	3	
__ brittle or ridged nails	0	1	2	3	
__ difficult elimination with tense colon	0	1	2	3	Total Score
__ lack of sense of direction in life	0	1	2	3	of AdditsymptLv
__ fear of making decisions	0	1	2	3	symptoms ....

Intake form for the research project *Acupuncture in the Treatment of Depression*   ©1999–2000, Rosa N. Schnyer

For Client to Complete

Last 2 weeks!

	Absent	Mild	Moderate	Severe	For acupuncturist to complete
AdditsymptHt					
__ excitement causes heat or perspiration	0	I	2	3	
__ burning sensitivity or irritation of mouth, tongue,	0	I	2	3	
urethra, vagina, anus	0	I	2	3	Total Score
__ frequent urination or bowel movements from nervousness	0	I	2	3	of AdditsymptHt
__ palpitations when nervous, upset, exhausted	0	I	2	3	symptoms ....
AdditsymptSp					
__ craving for sweets	0	I	2	3	
__ lingering hunger after meals	0	I	2	3	
__ hard to gain, lose or regulate weight	0	I	2	3	
__ easily worried	0	I	2	3	
__ difficulty focusing	0	I	2	3	
__ overwhelmed by details, upset by changes	0	I	2	3	
__ feelings of guilt	0	I	2	3	Total Score
__ obsessive thinking	0	I	2	3	of AdditsymptSp
__ phobias	0	I	2	3	symptoms ....
AdditsymptLu					
__ frequent colds or coughs	0	I	2	3	
__ frequent runny nose or stuffy sinuses	0	I	2	3	
__ itchiness or rashes of skin	0	I	2	3	
__ easily disappointed or offended	0	I	2	3	
__ sensitive to wind, cold or dryness	0	I	2	3	
__ sadness/tendency to weep	0	I	2	3	Total Score
__ easily affected negatively by others' problems	0	I	2	3	of AdditsymptLu
__ melancholic/nostalgic for the past	0	I	2	3	symptoms ....
AdditsymptKd					
__ weak or sore knees, ankles, feet	0	I	2	3	
__ forgetfulness	0	I	2	3	
__ puffiness or swelling of feet and ankles	0	I	2	3	
__ puffiness around eyes	0	I	2	3	
__ dull or diminished hearing	0	I	2	3	
__ low humming in ears	0	I	2	3	
__ easily disgruntled	0	I	2	3	
__ lack of willpower, drive, initiative	0	I	2	3	
__ hopelessness/despair/feeling aimless	0	I	2	3	Total Score
__ rigid mental attitude	0	I	2	3	of AdditsymptKd
__ great exhaustion/no willpower	0	I	2	3	symptoms ....

Intake form for the research project *Acupuncture in the Treatment of Depression*

Describe your menstrual periods or the general pattern:

Duration: How many days does it last? _____

Menarche: How old were you when you first got your period? _____

Date of beginning of last menstrual period: _____

Have you taken Birth Control Pills? _____

Regularity:
___ regular, every ..... (28, 30, 35) days
___ irregular, tends to be early
___ irregular, tends to be late
___ irregular, sometimes early, sometimes late

Color, consistency and volume:
___ pale red
___ dark red
___ rusty
___ bright red
___ begins dark red, becomes bright red
___ begins bright red, becomes dark red
___ mixed with dark clots
___ few clots
___ larger and a lot of clots
___ excessive flow
___ scant flow
___ begins scanty, becomes excessive
___ inconsistent flow (stops and starts and stops)

Pain:
___ precedes period, relieved by flow
___ associated with passing clots
___ with distension and bloating
___ after period
___ diffuse cramping
___ sharp and piercing
___ fixed in location
___ resists pressure
___ feels better with pressure
___ better with heat
___ better with movement
___ worse with movement
___ worse with lack of movement
___ better with rest
___ localized on the lower abdomen, sides of
abdomen, lower back, legs

Premenstrual symptoms:
___ breast distension
___ sharp breast pain
___ abdominal distension
___ water retention
___ cravings (salt, sweets, chocolate, other)
___ pain in low back, sacrum, hips
___ achy joints
___ need to sleep a lot
___ more difficulty sleeping
___ significant changes in emotions

Other:
___ fibroids
___ ovarian cysts
___ endometriosis
___ fibrocystic breasts
___ tubal ligation
___ miscarriages
___ pregnancies
___ infertility

COMMENTS specific to the menstrual cycle or the reproductive system:

_____
_____
_____
_____
_____
_____
_____
_____
_____
_____
_____
_____
_____

1. What is most stressful to you in your life at the moment?

2. What emotion are you experiencing primarily at this time? (Anger, frustration, worry, fear, sorrow, lack of joy, others)

3. With what emotion do you handle yourself outwardly? Do you think people perceive you as you feel?

4. How do you feel about yourself? About your relationships? About your job?

About myself:

About my relationships:

About my job:

5. What do you like the most about yourself?

What do you dislike the most about yourself?

6. What is it about your day to day life that is most satisfying, most frustrating, most difficult, most easy?

most satisfying: most difficult:

most frustrating: most easy:

7. What concept, principle or metaphor has been the motivating force in your life that has propelled you and inspired you?

List the 3 main physical symptoms and the 3 main emotional/mental symptoms that characterize your depression at this time:

PHYSICAL: MENTAL/EMOTIONAL:

1.   1.

2.   2.

3.   3.

Practitioner's assessment

Client Initials: _____

Client ID #: _____

Today's Date: _____

PULSE

Acupuncturist: _____

1		2		3		4
Fast	**Slow**	**Floating**	**Deep**	**Has force**	**Has no force**	**Other qualities**
Fast	Slow	Floating	Deep	Has force	Has no force	Wiry
Skipping	Choppy	Vacuous	Weak	Replete	Weak	Slippery
Racing	Relaxed	Soft/soggy	Hidden	Tight	Fine	Long
Stirring	Bound	Hollow	Confined	Large	Vacuous	Short
	Regularly intermittent	Surging		Faint	Soggy/soft	
		Scattered			Hidden	
		Drumskin				

Rate: _____   Overall Quality: _____

Outstanding pulse: _____

Right		
Cun	Guan	Chi

Left		
Cun	Guan	Chi

Comments: _____

_____

TONGUE

Body

Shape _____

Color _____

Moisture _____

Movement _____

Cracks _____

Coating

Shape _____

Color _____

Moisture _____

OBSERVATION:

Overall impression:

Shen: Facial Color (overall/eyes, mouth):   Voice:

Body form: Hands: Other:

SUMMARY

TONGUE:

PALPATION:

Pulse Picture

Mu Points   **Shu Points**   **Three Heaters**

Meridians and Zones   **Hara**

Patient profile

1. Differentiate the Signs and Symptoms (including main symptoms and symptoms associated with depression).
2. Remember that based on this framework the patterns of disharmony are constructed by evaluating the degree of involvement of four features:
   i) Qi stagnation
   ii) Shen disturbance
   iii) Vacuity of qi/yang and/or repletion of dampness/phlegm
   iv) Vacuity of yin/blood and/or repletion of heat/fire
3. NAME YOUR PATTERNS BY USING THE PATTERN NAMES USED IN THE BOX BELOW AND MANUAL.
4. If needed, describe the disease mechanism to clarify further.

Qi stagnation	Shen disturbance	Qi/yang vacuity	Yin repletion: dampness/phlegm	Blood/yin vacuity	Yang repletion and vacuity heat
Liver depression Qi stagnation	Ht blood vacuity	VacQi–Sp	Spvac–dampaccum	Bloodvac–Lv	Stagnation–heat (see qistag column)
Stagnation Ht/Lu	Hi qi vacuity	VacYang–Sp	Phlegm obstructing the heart	Yinvac Lv Kd Lu	Hyperactivity of liver yang
Stagnation–heat	Ht yin vacuity	VacQi–Lu	Phlegm fire harassing the heart		Liver fire
	Yin vacuity, fire effulgence (vacuity heat)	VacQi–Kd	Phlegm dampness obstruction and stagnation		Liver fire with dampness Damp–heat
	Repletion: Qi stagnation Ht/Lu	VacYang–Kd			Vacuity heat
	Depressive heat affecting Ht/Lu				
	Heart fire				
	Phlegm obstructing the heart				
Blood stasis	Phlegm fire harassing the heart		Observe if dampness is combined with heat (damp–heat)		Yin fire

Pattern(s) Differentiation:

(Complex) Pattern

Treatment Principles:

Summary sheet for data tabulation

Note to the assessing acupuncturist: when conducting your evaluation and reviewing the intake form, rate the severity of each presenting pattern 0–3, as described in the adjacent box. In addition, establish your treatment principles based on the priority of the patterns presented. Take into consideration both the severity and the number of symptoms present for each category, the additional/overlapping symptoms, as well as the signs (i.e. tongue and pulse).

Rating of Severity

0 absent

1 mild (infrequent or not intense)

2 moderate (frequent or more intense)

3 severe (constant or very intense)

	Qi stagnation	Shen disturbance	Qi/yang vacuity	Yin repletion: dampness/ phlegm	Blood/yin vacuity	Yang repletion and vacuity heat	Additional symptoms by organ
Specific pattern	__ LvQiStag __ LvQiStag–Lu/Ht __ LvQiStag–Heat		__ Qivac–Sp __ Yangvac–Sp __ Qivac–Lu __ Qivac–Kd		__ Bloodvac–Lv __ Yinvac	__ Vacuityheat __ Yan Repletion	__ Lv __ Lu __ Ht __ Sp __ Kd
Total score in symptom category	__ /66 = __ %	__ /42 = __ %	__ /66 = __ %	__ /48 = __ %	__ /39 = __ %	__ /39 = __ %	
Additional/ overlapping signs & symptoms							
Pulse							
Tongue							
Overall rating for this disease category							

Intake form for the research project *Acupuncture in the Treatment of Depression*   ©1999–2000, Rosa N. Schnyer

Rating of patient suitability

After completing the assessment, please rate the suitability of the patient for acupuncture treatment.

Category	Not Present				Very Prominent
■ Phlegm obstructing the heart	1	2	3	4	5
■ Phlegm fire harassing the heart	1	2	3	4	5
■ Blood stasis	1	2	3	4	5
■ Severe or long-standing vacuity	1	2	3	4	5
■ Severe history of psychosocial stress and trauma	1	2	3	4	5
	Very Unsuitable				Very Suitable
Global Rating of Suitability	1	2	3	4	5

Rating Considerations:

Two main patterns might render the patient less suitable for treatment by acupuncture alone:

■ The presence of phlegm obstructing the heart, phlegm fire harassing the heart, and blood stasis as the primary patterns of disharmony or as very significant components

■ The presence of severe and long-standing vacuity of either yin or yang.

These patterns are best treated by a combination of acupuncture and Chinese botanical medicine, and dietary and behavioral changes, and are most recalcitrant to acupuncture alone. Our hypothesis is that the level of severity for these patterns correlates to chronic and recurrent depression, double depression, or depression superimposed upon another axis I disorder. It is our interest to explore whether people who present a clearly defined depressive episode, based on traditional Western measures using our exclusion criteria, do in fact fall mostly on patterns of disharmony that exclude those patterns mentioned above.

In addition, an extensive history of psychosocial stress and trauma that has not been previously explored by the patient, through psychotherapy or other means, might render acupuncture insufficient in the treatment of depression. In these cases, our hypothesis is that acupuncture and psychotherapy combined will give better and more lasting results. We are interested as well to explore whether acupuncture treatment alone prompts in the patient the 'need' or 'desire' to explore a history of psychosocial stressors, or facilitates the psychological process.

Appendix B

Pulse Definitions

1		2		3		4
Fast	**Slow**	**Floating**	**Deep**	**Has force**	**Has no force**	**Other qualities**
Fast	Slow	Floating	Deep	Has force	Has no force	Wiry
Skipping	Choppy	Vacuous	Weak	Replete	Weak	Slippery
Racing	Relaxed	Soft/soggy	Hidden	Tight	Fine	Long
Stirring	Bound	Hollow	Confined	Large	Vacuous	Short
	Regularly intermittent	Surging		Faint	Soggy/soft	
		Scattered			Hidden	
		Drumskin				

Fast: above 90 beats per minute

Fast pulses:
1. **Skipping:** rapid, irregularly interrupted
2. **Racing:** very rapid, over 120 beats per minute
3. **Stirring:** slippery, rapid, forceful

Slow: below 60 beats per minute

Slow pulses:
1. **Choppy:** slow, relaxed, stagnant, fine, small, short, slows down and speeds up; seems to lose a beat but then recovers
2. **Relaxed/moderate:** on the verge of slow, relaxed, loose, slack
3. **Bound:** slow, relaxed, stops at irregular intervals

Floating/superficial: can be felt with light pressure; as pressure increases it disappears. When pressure is released, it regains full strength

Floating pulses
1. **Vacuous:** slow, floating, large, forceless; also general term for various forceless pulses
2. **Soft/soggy:** floating, fine, soft, forceless
3. **Hollow/scallion:** floating, soft, large body but empty center
4. **Surging:** floating, large; comes on exuberant, departs debilitated
5. **Scattered:** floating, large, without root; it becomes changeable even with light pressure, becoming chaotic; with heavier pressure, it disappears
6. **Drumskin:** floating, large, wiry, with an empty center

Deep: can be felt only with heavy pressure; cannot be felt with moderate or light pressure

Deep pulses:
1. **Weak:** deep, fine, forceless, soft
2. **Hidden:** difficult to feel, close to the bone; not large or strong
3. **Confined:** deep, large, wiry, forceful, strong

Has force:

Pulses that have force:
1. **Replete:** long, wiry, large, hard, replete, has a surplus; may be floating or deep; also used as a general term for forceful pulses
2. **Tight:** has strength, it is long and it is not fine; stronger and bigger than wiry

Has no force:

Pulses that have no force:
1. **Weak:** see above
2. **Fine:** soft, weak, without strength but persistent; it is continuous and not scattered by pressure
3. **Vacuous:** see above
4. **Soggy/soft:** see above
5. **Faint:** very, very fine and forceless
6. **Hidden:** see above

Other:
1. **Wiry:** fine, long, has strength
2. **Slippery:** comes smoothly floating and uninhibited
3. **Short:** does not fill its location longitudinally
4. **Long:** can be felt beyond its own location

Source: Flaws (1995).

Appendix C

Developing an Acupuncture Treatment Manual To Use in Clinical Trials

The development of treatment protocols that can be used reliably in clinical trials of acupuncture requires systematic articulation of both the theoretical framework and the selection of treatment strategies and techniques. In order to conform to the rigor of established research methodology and yet maintain fidelity to acupuncture as a medical system, it is necessary to deliver replicable and standardized treatments that allow for an individualized approach. By developing a treatment manual it is possible to attain standardization and maintain replicability, while at the same time provide individually tailored treatments based on a differential diagnosis that reflects the particular acupuncture style chosen.

Over the course of six years, the manual we developed originally has been modified substantially to provide a more detailed and well-specified articulation of the approach. Additionally, as needed, the protocol has been adapted and modified to address the characteristics specific to each population targeted in different studies, as articulated in Chapter 4 under 'Depression and The Life Cycle'. In order to illustrate the essential components, and the process we followed in manualizing the acupuncture protocol, we have outlined here the features characteristic of the original treatment manual used in the pilot study described on Chapter 7.

1. The essential features of the approach:

- An assumption that Western-defined depression is heterogeneous and may be characterized by one or more distinct patterns of disharmony, which may differ for different clients with depression.

- Emphasis on the eight guiding criteria, viscera and bowels, and qi, blood and body fluids as the basis for assessment and treatment.

- The use of standard CM evaluation tools including interview, pulse assessment and tongue observation.

- The use of the step-by-step methodology characteristic of eight-principle pattern differentiation, (differentiation of signs and symptoms, establishment of disease mechanisms, patterns and combinations, outline of treatment principles, and selection of treatment plan).

- Extensive use of the five phases in the initial interview to determine constitutional characteristics.

- Palpation of the abdomen and channels for point selection.

- Comprehensive consideration of the channel system in treatment design.

- A goal of producing clinically meaningful change: improved balance rather than disharmony, remission as defined by DSM-IV criteria, and Hamilton Rating Scale for Depression (HRSD) score ≤ 6.

2. Duration and optimal frequency

Acute treatments to be delivered twice per week for eight weeks, and once per week for four weeks. Ideally, we would suggest adding maintenance and continuation treatments semi-monthly and then monthly for the next year.

3. Methodology

Following intake screening by telephone, and a structured clinical face-to-face interview to establish patient suitability (see point 5 below), participants were assessed monthly by interview, and weekly using self report measures, while in the study. Trained clinical raters blind to treatment status conducted assessment during the treatment phase.

4. Adaptations or modifications

The treatment was tailored to address depression in women aged 18–45. Treatments were tailored according to the phases of the menstrual cycle, in accordance with the principles of Chinese Medicine (see Chapter 4). In those women who were no longer menstruating, treatment was adjusted accordingly. In subsequent studies, treatments were tailored to address the needs of the different populations that were targeted in each study; the protocol was adapted to women during pregnancy and postpartum, men and women in ages ranging from 18–65.

5. Patient suitability

Suitability for participation in each study was determined on the basis of specific criteria for inclusion in each study, outlined in the box on page 211.

6. Characteristics that differentiate this approach from others

The protocol developed for use in the clinical trial, was based exclusively on an eight-principle pattern differentiation and employed acupuncture exclusively. Although we did evaluate the constitutional predisposition of clients within a five-phase framework, we did not use five phase based treatment strategies as part of our treatment protocol. Furthermore, although we acknowledged and incorporated the complexity of the channel system in point selection, we tailored our treatments exclusively on the use of the 14 Main Channels.

7. Clinical experience and empirical support

The clinical experience and formal training of RNS formed the basis for the development of the manual.

Inclusion Criteria

- Age 16–60
- Meets the DSM-IV diagnostic criteria for current Major Depression. In the course of the Structured Clinical Interview for DSM (SCID-P; Spitzer et al 1990), she must experience for a period of at least 2 weeks in which at least 5 of the following symptoms have been present and represent a change from a previous level of functioning; at least 1 of the 5 symptoms must be either #1 (depressed mood) or #2 (loss of interest or pleasure):

  1. Depressed mood most of the day, nearly every day.
  2. Markedly diminished interest or pleasure in all or almost all activities, most of the day, nearly every day.
  3. Significant weight loss or weight gain (>5%) when not dieting; or decrease or increase in appetite nearly every day.
  4. Insomnia or hypersomnia nearly every day.
  5. Psychomotor Agitation or Retardation nearly every day.
  6. Fatigue or loss of energy nearly every day.
  7. Feelings of worthlessness or excessive or inappropriate guilt (which may be delusional) nearly every day.
  8. Diminished ability to think or concentrate, or indecisiveness, nearly every day.
  9. Recurrent thoughts of death or suicide.

- Symptoms cause clinically significant distress or impairment.

Exclusion Criteria

- Symptoms must not be the direct physiological effects of a substance or a general medical condition
- Symptoms must not be a normal reaction to the death of a loved one (Uncomplicated Bereavement)
- Symptoms do not meet criteria for dysthymia, chronic major depression, bipolar depression
- There is not the presence of any other current Axis I diagnosis besides Major Depressive Disorder
- There is no history of psychosis or mania
- There has been no substance abuse or dependence within the past 4 months
- There is no current treatment for depression (including counselling, psychotherapy, pharmacotherapy, Alcoholics Anonymous, or support groups)
- There are no endocrine abnormalities
- There is no history of CNS lesions or any medical disorder or treatment that could cause depression
- There is not active suicidal potential necessitating immediate treatment.
- If a woman, she is not pregnant.

8. Theoretical framework and theoretical references

As detailed in Chapter 3.

9. Etiology of depression according to Chinese Medicine

As detailed in Chapter 4.

10. Assessment of depression according to Chinese Medicine

As detailed in Chapters 4 and 5.

11. Strategies and techniques

As detailed in Chapter 5.

12. Implementation of the assessment framework

As detailed in Chapter 5.

13. Treatment delivery

As detailed in Chapter 5.

14. Dealing with acute symptoms

As detailed in Chapter 8. Additionally a list of telephone crisis and contact numbers was provided to clients listing the Principal Investigator, the Project Administrator, the crisis coverage for the study and general crisis counseling in the metropolitan area.

15. Case histories

As detailed in Chapter 6.

16. Assessment tools

As detailed in Appendix A.

Index